Surviving your Placement in Health and Social Care: A Student handbook

Surviving your Placement in Health and Social Care:
A student handbook

Joan Healey and Margaret Spencer

Open University Press

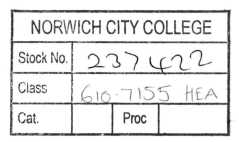

Open University Press
McGraw-Hill Education
McGraw-Hill House
Shoppenhangers Road
Maidenhead
Berkshire
England
SL6 2QL

email: enquiries@openup.co.uk
world wide web: www.openup.co.uk

and Two Penn Plaza, New York, NY 10121—2289, USA

First published 2008

A catalogue record of this book is available from the British Library

ISBN-10: 0-33-522259-5 (pb) 0-33-522260-9 (hb)
ISBN-13: 978-0-33-522259-9 (pb) 978-0-33-522260-5 (hb)

Library of Congress Cataloging-in-Publication Data
CIP data applied for

Typeset by Kerrypress Ltd, Luton, Bedfordshire
Printed and bound in the UK by Bell and Bain Ltd, Glasgow

The McGraw·Hill Companies

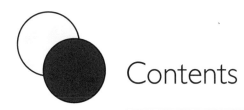

Contents

Dedicated to Bridie, Tom and Kate

Acknowledgements: To Mum and Dad who always believed I could, to Phil without whom it would not have been possible, and to Keith Shelton who facilitated the life changing decision

Margaret

1 Using this book

- **Read this chapter before you start**
- **Use of terminology**
- **Using this book**
- **Chapter outcomes**

Read this chapter before you start

> By the end of this chapter you will be able to:
>
> ➡ explore what is on offer in this book
> ➡ identify your needs and prioritize them
> ➡ decide in which order you will work through this book
> ➡ set a realistic framework which identifies dates and times for each chapter you need
> ➡ feel a sense of purpose and control.

The reason for writing this book is to help you through your placements. It is aimed at all health and social care professionals, whether it is your first placement or last placement or indeed any in between. It could also be used to bridge the gap between your pre-registration course and your first job. It includes all the things that we go through in our prep sessions and, we are sure, all the things that your own lecturers will go through in yours. We go through all the issues again when we visit the students on placement, and again when anyone is failing a placement. People listen at the time and then go home, get involved with flatmates, partners, or children and then when they have the opportunity to reflect often think, 'Mmmm what did they say again about ...?' If this is you, read on.

This book is different in that if you drift off when someone is talking and miss that vital ten minutes during which the crucial piece of information was relayed you can not go back. With this book you can plan your time and at your leisure read and re-read the information and make sense of it in your own time, when the time is right for you to be fully receptive and alert to your own development.

Use of terminology

We are aware there are many different terms for the role of the person who educates you in practice, including: supervisors, mentors, practice placement educators, practice teacher and clinical tutors. We have decided, for ease of reading, to use the term 'educator' throughout this book, so whenever this generic word is used it is intended to cover all those individual roles. We also mention clients, patients and service users. Choose whichever one suits you and your situation at the time.

We have deliberately tried to demystify some of the theory which underpins education in practice. This does not mean that it ceases to exist but once you understand the basics you can begin to explore the terminology and theory for yourself. As with other terminology, for ease of reading, we have decided to use the term 'learning objectives' throughout this book, although you may be more familiar with the term 'learning outcomes'.

Many other books talk about educational theories; we have made some suggestions for further reading at the end of each chapter so that you can find out about these theories in more detail. Then, if you want to or need to, you will be able to review more of the literature that exists about, for instance, learning outcomes and objectives, and come to your own conclusions about which is most appropriate for you. You will be able to identify the historical developments that have occurred socially and politically to enable changes in terminology from 'patients' to 'service users' etc., and how this has impacted on your own profession.

Using this book

All that comes later … in this book we are talking directly to you and when you write down your answers to our self-assessment questions, you are answering us back. As we are not in the room with you as you work through the questions, you can be as honest as you like: only you will know the answers to the questions. Being a health and social care professional in any area poses challenges and requires you to make changes in your behaviour and attitudes during your time at university. This will stop and start as you work through the course, and sometimes you will notice many changes in yourself and other times none at all. Placements are often a time when you are challenged personally and professionally and, as a result, these are often the times of most rapid change.

You have chosen to be on a health and social care course, and because of this choice you will have to go on placement to demonstrate that you are competent, and eventually receive your state registration. Hopefully, this book will help you through the placement process. But, like passing placements, it will only help if you fully engage in the process. That means being active and not passive. If you complete the exercises as you go along you will gain much more from this book than simply reading it alone. By selecting this book you have made a positive step forward in becoming a health and social care professional.

Coming on a course that involves working with people all day every day, will require you to look at yourself and reflect continually in order to try and improve what you have done and get better at what you are going to do. It is easier and safer to start that process in the comfort of your own home, at a time of your choosing. You may wish to work through this book with a small group of other students, the choice is yours.

Being a health and social care professional requires reflection and evidence of continual personal and professional development, not just throughout the course but throughout the rest of your professional career in order to remain state registered. If personal development and change fills you with excitement, enthusiasm, and motivation you are on the right course.

Remember we talked about engaging in the process? Well, that starts now. This symbol ⬯ is an indication that you need to think about an issue and write down your thoughts about it. It is essential that you do this – and you can always use it as evidence of development in your continuing professional development file, especially if you are able to repeat the process later in the course or your career. It is intended that working through this book will be a dynamic process.

Box 1.1 ⬯

Getting started

Make sure you have 10–15 minutes to carry out the next exercise.

Imagine you have numbers 1–10 to award yourself: 10/10 means you are confident and competent, 1/10 means you have not quite started on this yet and do not even know what the title means. Try to put a different number on each line. This will help you think through what is involved on a placement, how much you know or do not know about it, and how much time you will need to allocate to each area in preparation before you go on placement or during placement if you are already there.

1–10

Preparing personally for placement	
Reflecting on your behaviour	
Writing learning outcomes	
Self-assessment	

Making complex decisions using your professional reasoning skills	
Work/life balance and time management	
Using supervision	
Knowledge of working with other professionals – where you fit in the jigsaw	
Keeping a record of your progress personally and professionally (portfolios and progress files)	
Evidence-based practice	

Great, this is an impressive start and you have already demonstrated that you can reflect, self-assess, and prioritize.

This ranking will provide you with an opportunity to begin to think about what preparation you need to do before your next placement. It also will give you a reasonable idea about which area you need to tackle first.

Box 1.2

Now re-write the areas that you have marked out of ten below, starting with 1/10 and working your way up to 10/10. This would probably be the best order for you to work through this book. If you have another way that you think would work better for you, then write that in.

Topic	Book chapter

It is impossible to tackle all of this list at once and is probably unachievable and counterproductive anyway. So you need to think about your time and start to use it wisely. What are your current priorities, and how much time can you allocate to each chapter or topic? How much time do you have before you go on your next placement or are you already on it?

On a placement you will have to allocate time to each client or group including any preparation, note writing and travel, etc. Although this is a little flexible, you need to be able to start developing the ability to identify how long things will take you. As a beginner things always take longer as everything is new, so you have to factor that in. Have a look at your diary. If you have not got one yet now is the time to get one as it is essential.

   Which chapter received 1/10?

This chapter topic is obviously a priority and will take you longer to work through. Start with an hour and see how you progress. Have a look through your diary and decide when would be the best time for you to start on this chapter. Write it in your diary, so you can start as you mean to go on. Setting realistic dates and times to work through each chapter will hopefully enable you to use this book to its full advantage, and develop some good working strategies along the way.

Good luck on your placement! We hope you will find the chapters in this book valuable.

Chapter outcomes

Now that you have completed this chapter you should feel more confident to:

➡ use this book more effectively to meet your personal needs
➡ identify your needs and prioritize them
➡ decide in which order you will work through this book
➡ set a realistic framework which identifies dates and times for each chapter you need
➡ feel a sense of purpose and control.

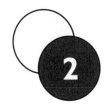

2 Preparing yourself for the placement experience

- **Preparing yourself for the placement experience**
- **Learning about yourself from feedback**
- **Preparing yourself for emotional challenges**
- **Some guidelines for dealing with the emotional aspects of placements**
- **Your educator and you**
- **The service and you: practicalities**

By the end of this chapter you will be able to:

➡ evaluate your existing skills
➡ explore how to use constructive feedback
➡ consider how to prepare yourself for the emotional challenges of placement
➡ be clear about the relationship between you, the service user and the service you are providing.

Preparing yourself for the placement experience

While you are at university you could say that only part of your personality is on display and that part is mostly you as 'the student'. At university it is primarily your theoretical knowledge that is assessed. Your tutors perhaps know only a small amount about you as a person, but much more about your knowledge and ability to convey that knowledge: when you step into a placement things change. On placement you are asked to act as a professional and, in some ways, everything about you is being assessed. The way you present yourself to other people, including how you dress and the way you communicate with others; the empathy and understanding you show to the service users; your ability to organize yourself – all these things will be part of your placement assessment. This can be a shock to new students and is something that is worth thinking about before each placement. Some of the things you learn about yourself on placement may well change your whole idea of yourself.

In order to prepare yourself for your placement experience, you will need to think about several key things:

yourself

(?) What constitutes your comfort zone and what sort of things are outside of that?

(?) How self-aware are you?

(?) What are your strengths and your development needs?

the service users you may be working with

(?) Why are they likely to be using the service?

(?) What do you need to know about their situations and what they may be going through?

the service

(?) What are the expectations of you as a student?

(?) What might your 'employers' be asking you to do?

Box 2.1

Starting with you!

It is always a useful idea to begin with a base line. A self-rating scale of where you think you are currently at, can help with this. It may help if you start by looking at the following areas and rate where you think your skills are at the moment. You can use these self-rating scales all the way through your training as they can help you monitor how you are developing. However, a rating scale on its own will only be of limited use and you can take it further by setting yourself some objectives and an action plan about how you are going to address these. This will link in really well with your personal and professional portfolio and placement learning objectives.

Ratings:

❶ I feel really unsure of my skills in this area
❷ I feel a little unsure of my skills in this area

❸ I feel I have some skills in this area
❹ I feel I have some good skills in this area
❺ I feel very confident about my skills in this area

Try to rate yourself for the following categories and the sub-skills within each one.

Skill	Rating 1–5
Communication – verbal	
one-to-one with peers	
one-to-one with 'authority figures'	
in group settings with peers	
in group settings with colleagues	
Listening skills	
one-to-one with peers	
one-to-one with 'authority figures'	
in group settings	
Communication – non-verbal	
my own	
reading other people's	
How I present to others	
confidence with friends	
confidence with colleagues	
confidence with 'authority figures'	
assertiveness with friends	
assertiveness with colleagues	
assertiveness with 'authority figures'	

As a matter of interest why not ask someone you know to rate you as well. How does their rating compare with your own?

If you score below a **3** in any of the areas then they may be starting points for your learning objectives on placement. See Chapter 4 on learning objectives and how to write them to help you take this further.

Learning about yourself from feedback

At times throughout your placement it is likely that you will receive feedback about your behaviour or how you appear to other people, other staff, service users and carers. Much of this is bound to be positive but some may be more difficult to accept. How you react to this feedback will be crucial in determining how you learn from it. No one likes having to hear less than positive things about themselves and unless your educator is a very strange person, no-one finds it easy giving negative feedback, so it will not usually be done lightly. You can choose to react in several ways:

➡ **dismiss it** because you know you are not like that
➡ **get angry** with the person for saying it
➡ **ignore it** because you do not want to deal with it
➡ **accept it at face value** and think about what it means
➡ **accept it but check it out** with other people to see if it is what they think too.

The way you choose to respond will determine what and how you learn from the feedback you are given. Think about how you currently react if someone gives you some less than positive feedback and think about how you might prefer to react in the future, to ensure you make the most of your feedback.

Example 1

Julian is a first year nursing student on a placement in a busy cardiac ward in a large teaching hospital. His mentor has brought up the issue of his non-verbal communication in a supervision session and reports that several of the staff have commented on how disinterested or bored he appears at handovers. This shocks Julian as he actually finds the handovers interesting. He looks forward to hearing about how the patients have been but so far he has not been asked to contribute. His mentor is very kind about this feedback and says she should have told him to join in whenever he felt he had something to say and that she will encourage him to do this in the future. She does reiterate to him, however, that his body stance and non-verbal communication can make people think he is disinterested and she asks him to think about it.

How would you feel if someone said this about you? You may feel very upset or angry. People often interpret or confuse criticism of behaviour with criticism of them as a person. You may feel they are making assumptions about you from how you appear and this may feel unfair. Think about this yourself and remember how easy it is to make assumptions about people you do not know just from their appearance. Your educator does not know you as your friends do. She or he cannot interpret your behaviour in the light of their knowledge of you as a person as they do not have that information. They are trying to understand your behaviour. By giving you this feedback they are giving you a gift. Now you know how you were perceived to be by this person on that occasion. If you did not mean to be seen like that then what can you do about it?

Example 1, cont.

Julian is left with some choices now. He knows he is interested so surely she is wrong, but why would other people say that? He goes home that evening and talks to his friends about this. Most of them try to support him and say the mentor is just being picky and that things are very formal on acute wards. What his friends are saying is that it is the mentor's fault and not his. One of them, however, does point out that he does slump in his chair a lot and stare out of windows when maybe he is thinking. Julian asks the others about this and they agree that maybe he does do this sometimes.

On return to the placement the next day, Julian makes a point of looking at other people's non-verbal communication compared to his own and he has to admit that when he sits normally he does look quite different from the others in the group. He makes an extra effort to sit up more, make eye contact and contribute to discussions. At the next supervision session his mentor reports that colleagues have been remarking how much he has contributed this week.

Julian had a choice here about whether to think and act on the feedback or dismiss it. You too may well be in a similar situation at some point in your placement learning and you will have to decide what to do with the feedback.

It is not easy to receive critical feedback and it may cause us to get upset or angry but it is worth remembering that the feedback is about behaviour at a certain place, at a certain point in time and it is not a judgement of you as a person. It has the potential to lead to positive developments depending on how you react to it.

Preparing yourself for emotional challenges

You and the service user

The people using the services you will be going into have all been through some turmoil of some sort, whether this is because of physical illness, a mental health need or a social need. They will be going through an experience which is out of the ordinary run of things for them. This can range from a minor injury causing minor disruption to their lives, to a major crisis which has thrown their whole lives and future into question. As a professional who will be responsible for providing part of the service to them you will have to be able to cope with the potential emotional consequences of this on them and, possibly, their families and friends.

It can be daunting for a student to go out on a placement and be faced with working with people who are extremely upset and hurt about what they are going through, and you will need to think about how you are able to deal with that in some way. When you read someone's medical or social care notes before you go and see them for the first time, what goes through your mind? Your decisions on how much you engage with the emotional side of what people are going through may well be determined by your role but will also be influenced by your own emotional well-being. One way in which to prepare yourself for placement is to read fictional accounts and autobiographies which are about illness, or social issues. Here, in the *story* of what has happened comes the *meaning*, that is what these things mean to people. By doing this rather than just being armed with a set of facts (the theory), you can begin to engage with what it might mean to someone, for example, to be diagnosed with schizophrenia or become homeless or live with Parkinson's disease.

Example 2

You are a diagnostic radiographer student taking the next referral for someone with multiple fractures following a road traffic accident. You may know that you only have so many minutes to spend with this patient so it would be inappropriate to engage with the person about what they are going through. In spite of this, however, you can convey understanding and empathy just by a kind voice and a warm smile; by not rushing them, making sure they are as comfortable as possible; by conveying your human concern and warmth towards them.

Example 3

You are a physiotherapist student meeting someone for their first outpatient appointment who has severe hand injuries following a fire. You know from her notes that she lost her partner in the fire and that because of her injuries she is struggling to cope with looking after her two small children. Do you just focus on the injury or do you talk to her about what she has been through? Do you feel you have the skills to be able to do this? Do you have the time in the appointment to do this? These are the questions you can ask yourself. Can you find a way of acknowledging the enormity of what she has to deal with while at the same time keeping focused on your role in her treatment? To do this, think about what it makes you feel. Are you scared at the thought of mentioning it? Do you think she might become upset if you ask her about it? Do you think you might become upset if she tells you about it? If you can convey to her your concern as another human being as well as being a professional who is going to help with some part of those problems, then you will be meeting her needs and fullfilling your role and the expectations of you. You do not have to be a counsellor but if service users are going to engage in treatment with you they need to feel that you understand what they are going through and that you care about what has happened to them and what they want to happen next.

Some guidelines for dealing with the emotional aspects of placements

How can you put yourself in the shoes of the service user and think about what they might be feeling like now? Imagine it is you that has been through the injury or problems of the person you are dealing with.

- What would be your concerns and worries?

- What would you want from someone treating you or dealing with your situation?

- What would you want the student to say to you and how would you like them to talk to you?

- Are you seeing the situation from their point of view not just your own?

- Ask yourself what it might feel like for them to be walking into your department?

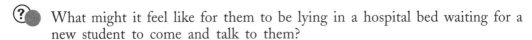

? What might it feel like for them to be lying in a hospital bed waiting for a new student to come and talk to them?

? What can you say or do to make people feel more at ease and to show them that you recognise the difficulties in their situation?

Starting by introducing yourself and saying why you are there will always put a person more at their ease. Remember that while you know what different uniforms mean, most other people do not. People may know what a physiotherapist or a nurse does but may not be so clear about the role of the social worker or the occupational therapist. It is up to you to explain why you are there.

Even something as simple as where you position yourself in relation to the person you are seeing can make a great deal of difference. Try to make sure that you are physically 'available' and there when the person comes into your office or department for the first time. Be there to greet them, making eye contact and shaking hands if that is appropriate. This conveys to the person that you are there for them. Give them your undivided attention. Do not try to finish your notes or tidy up while talking to them. This can make the person feel that you are too busy to see them and that you are not really interested. If you are going to someone's house to see them, wait to be invited in and to sit down. Take your cues from them. If you are going to someone's bedside, then make sure you pull up a chair if possible rather than standing above them, so that you are on an eye level with the person. This can give a more relaxed and equal start to the therapeutic relationship.

Think about *how* you acknowledge what they have been through in a simple statement and give them time to respond. You do not have to open up the issues any more and they may glide over the issues all together. You may take that as a cue that, for now, they do not wish to say any more or perhaps they might begin to tell you a little about how they are feeling and you can leave it at that for now.

How can you convey human warmth and care without becoming a counsellor?

➡ Keep your facial expressions and body language open.
➡ Show the person that they have your attention and that you are there for them.
➡ Acknowledge what you know they have been through from reading their notes or referral. It may be that you say something like this, 'It seems like you have had a lot going on over the last few months' or 'It seems like you've had a difficult time with this injury over the last few days' or 'It seems like you are going through a hard time with this illness'.
➡ Listen to how the person responds. If they answer yes or no only, you may want to leave it there. They may be telling you that they do not want to talk any further about it. If they say yes or no and then go on to tell you more, then listen and acknowledge what they are saying.

➡ If you are afraid that they will become upset or want to talk for a long time about what their problems are, then you can always bring it back to the reason you are there. At an opportune moment you can add that one of the reasons you are there is to try to alleviate the situation. Whatever your role is, whether you are the student nurse, social worker, radiographer, occupational therapist or physiotherapist, you are there to see if your intervention can make things better.

➡ Give the person the opportunity to talk and listen to what they say, acknowledging what they have said without questioning or taking it any further. Use non-verbal communication, nods and eye contact, to convey that you are listening and hearing what they are saying.

What can you do if someone becomes really upset and tearful?

Do not worry. There is nothing wrong with being upset and emotional in most cases. You have not caused this. It is the turmoil that the person has been going through that has caused this and the person has chosen to let out this emotion at this point. It can be frightening for a student and even for a lot of experienced professionals, but stay with it if you can. You can acknowledge what the person is saying and you do not have to be a knowledgeable counsellor to react as another caring human being: this is all that is required of you. If you feel the situation is too much for you, it is perfectly acceptable to fetch someone else who may be able to help you.

What do you do if you feel yourself getting upset?

Possibly everyone working in health and social care will become upset at what they see at some time. We are all human too and we are all service users at some point in our lives, as well as having friends and family who become services users at times. What we see our service users going through may well resonate with something you, or your friends or family have been through which may bring it all back to you. If you find yourself getting upset and tearful when you are with a service user it is usually best to take yourself out of the situation. This is because although it is understandable that at times we too can be upset, we are ultimately there for the service user not ourselves. It will not help the service user to think that they may, in some way, be upsetting you. They need to see that you are able to cope with what has happened to them and work with them to get through it. Explain to the person that you need to leave for a short while and, if necessary, fetch someone else to be with the person and take some time to compose yourself.

Supervision would be a really good place to discuss this with your educator/ mentor.

Your educator and you

One of the most frequently asked questions in preparation sessions for students before their first placement is, 'What do I do if I don't get on with my educator?' Your educator whether they be in radiography, occupational therapy, social work, nursing or physiotherapy, whatever their profession, will be expected to play a part in assessing your competence to practice. However, they are also there to facilitate your learning. Balancing this with assessing you while working alongside you everyday can make for a complex relationship. To complicate things even further still, you may find that you are invited out on team social occasions and then have to relate to your educator on another level as well.

If when you meet your educator you have the feeling that you may not get on, stop and ask yourself who they remind you of. Often it is the fact that they subconsciously remind us of someone else we have not got along with that makes us feel this way. If you can identify that you may be able to put it to one side and see the person for who they really are, not the person you are expecting them to be.

Learning styles

Sometimes you may find yourself placed with an educator who you think has a very different style to your own and wonder how you are going to get along. It is always a good idea to start with identifying your own learning styles and professional courses these days have a range of tools to help you do this. Your educator may have done this already for themselves. If they have not, then just asking them about what their preferred learning style is may encourage them to assess themselves.

We cannot guarantee that you will not have to work with someone with whom you have little in common and perhaps whose own style is the opposite of yours. This may often be the situation in your future workplace and how you deal with it now will help you develop the skills for doing this later on post-qualification.

What strategies could you think about for dealing with a situation like this if it happened to you on placement?

➡ Be as assertive as possible about your own learning style and needs while not criticizing your educator. Acknowledge the strengths of their learning style and your own.
➡ Ask your university tutor for support and advice and to check out your own perceptions of the situation.
➡ Look to other members of the staff team for support if possible; however, do not do this to undermine the educator but rather as additional support only.

➡ Write a reflective account of a supervision session as if you were the educator. What might they be thinking? How might the situation look from their point of view? What could this tell you about yourself and your educator?

Placement contracts

You have the right to expect certain levels of information and communication on placements to facilitate your learning and the educator should always be aware of these. To this end some placements and professions have placement contracts that agree some of these issues at the start of the placement. Here are some examples of issues that could be included in a placement contract between you and your educator. Even if you do not have a written contract to complete, it is worth using the following as a checklist for your first supervision session and to help you get the most out of your learning experience.

Checklist

- Have you both established your preferred learning styles?
- Do you have agreed learning objectives for the placement that you both sign up to?
- Have you agreed the boundaries of supervision – what topics are suitable, who sets the agenda, when and where it will be held?
- Do you both understand the same thing about how you will be assessed, when and where and who else may be consulted in the assessment?
- Do you have an agreed sense of what is expected of you in terms of assessment?
- Have you agreed practicalities around start and finish times, clothes/ uniforms, what to do if you are off sick, etc?
- Do you know what is expected of you week by week?

You cannot assume that you both understand something in the same way just because you have an assessment form. People can interpret things in different ways and, for example, what one educator understands about 'independent' may be different to what another understands by it. One educator may think if they go through with you what needs to be done in a certain situation and ask you to do it while watching from a distance, that this is 'independent'. Another may think that you need to identify what needs doing yourself and go off and do it, then report back to them and this is what constitutes being 'independent'. Make sure you have shared understandings.

If you feel that you have tried to find a shared understanding but cannot do this and if you feel that your educator is assessing you unfairly, you should always contact your link tutor from university who is there to support the process and can negotiate and mediate between you both. For more exploration of this topic, have a look at Chapter 8 on supervision.

The service and you: practicalities

Last but not least in this equation are the practicalities of your placement. Do not underestimate how important it is to establish some of the basic ground rules about practicalities. Think about how you make the first contact with your placement. Do you send a letter or make a phone call? Do they need you to send a CV and if so what should it include? This first communication will make the very important first impression and can help the placement educator to structure your induction. When you do start, something like arriving late is usually acceptable only as a one off or in special circumstances but can be construed as being unprofessional if it is habitual.

Practical tips

➡ Ask your educator for advice about any essential pre-placement reading. Do not just rely on university tutor advice about this as it needs to be tailored to your specific placement and educator who may be using a unique approach.
➡ Always travel to the placement and visit before you start, if at all practical. Doing this gives you an idea of travel time and means that you will not turn up late on the first day and possibly create a bad impression.
➡ Be prepared to be tired. You may well be travelling much more than you are used to and you will be on placement usually for a full day and over a full week. The pressure of being assessed on placement in itself can be stressful and add to the feeling of tiredness. The most common thing students say when they return from placement is, 'Why didn't you tell us it was going to be so tiring!' Make allowances for this if you can and look at your work/life balance (have a look at the Chapter 7 on time management).
➡ Make sure you establish any dress code or uniform policy, including issues around tattoos and body piercing, if they apply to you.

Practicalities are important! Get these things right and you will make that all important positive first impression. The rest will be easier if you can get off to a good start.

Chapter outcomes

Having read this chapter you should now:

➡ have a clearer view of your own skills and strengths
➡ be prepared to use feedback on your skills to develop further
➡ have a greater sense of the types of challenges you may face.

Further reading:

Alsop, A. and Ryan, S. (2001) *Making the most of fieldwork education: a practical approach.* 2nd edn. Cheltenham: Nelson Thornes Ltd.

Levett-Jones, T. ((2007) *The clinical placement: an essential guide for nursing students.* Edinburgh: Churchill Livingstone.

Shardlow, S. and Doel, M. (2002) *Learning to practice in social work.* London: Jessica Kingsley.

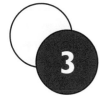

3 Reflective practice

- **What is reflective practice?**
- **Why is reflective practice so important to our learning and professional development?**
- **Reflection and critical reflection**
- **Reflective partners**
- **Writing up your reflections: some tips**
- **Critical incidents**
- **Models of reflection**

By the end of this chapter you will be able to:

➡ understand the importance of reflective practice in learning
➡ recognise the difference between reflection and critical reflection
➡ find a style of writing up reflections using the critical incident format and reflective journal
➡ recognize and choose between some of the most common reflective models.

What is reflective practice?

We see ourselves in many ways. For instance, one of those ways is to stand in front of a mirror and examine ourselves and what we look like physically. Other ways we find out about ourselves are when we ask friends about ourselves, for instance, 'What do I look like in this?' or 'Do you think I handled that ok?' You ask for feedback and information about yourself. Reflective practice is just a way of doing this and looking at our learning and professional development so it too involves putting ourselves in front of a mirror, inspecting what we do and how we do it. It can also involve others, asking them what they think of what we have done or even putting ourselves in their shoes and thinking about how they experienced what we did. The aim of it all is for us to gain a wider picture of ourselves and our practice from which we can learn. From this we can take forward the good things and do something about the things we do not like so much.

When we are engaging in reflection about ourselves, we try to look at something from lots of different angles and ask ourselves what happened, what went on and why. From asking ourselves those questions we can gain new insight into ourselves and our practice and identify ways in which we can develop to our full potential both personally and professionally. Obviously in order to do this we need to be receptive to new angles or visions of ourselves. We can choose to stand in front of a mirror and only see the surface, only see the good things, or we can look behind the surface and take on board the deeper elements that make up our image. We can move the mirror and see ourselves from different angles or we can put ourselves in a different light and we will appear differently. If we are prepared to open ourselves to this, then we can move on. We can become reflective practitioners and develop. If we choose to stay with the surface appearance we will not move forward.

The same applies to reflective practice: no-one can make you do this. You need to be ready and feel in a position of security and trust where you can allow yourself to question your own motives and practice. In order to be able to do this, the process of reflective practice can be divided into two:

❶ The personal reflections that you form yourself and choose to divulge or not: the raw material with which you can explore your practice further.
❷ The structured reflections that come from personal ones and can be used as the basis of supervision discussions and written up as evidence of your reflective abilities and professional development in your professional development portfolios.

In this chapter we will look at how to develop skills in both parts of the process.

Why is reflective practice so important to our learning and professional development?

We learn in many different ways. At university or college we may be studying in many different styles. For instance, sometimes you may be using a problem-based learning approach or using combinations of large lectures and smaller workshops or tutorials. You will find that perhaps one method suits you more than another. Learning on placement demands very different skills to that of learning in university. On placement you are asked both to use your knowledge and develop it at the same time, while working in real life situations where the consequences of your learning and professional knowledge and skills can directly affect the lives of vulnerable people. The complexity of the situations you will be working in demand that you synthesize a great deal of knowledge from university, simultaneously with knowledge and skills you have developed from placement (and previous placement experiences) and different colleagues. In the placement arena there are rarely easy answers. We approach every situation as a new one inasmuch as every person we deal with will be an individual with specific and individual needs. We learn in practice from hypothesizing from our knowledge, from experience, and from evidence and we attempt best practice for a given situation and a given individual. As we gain more experience this knowledge and skill base expands and we can apply it usefully in another comparable situation. Reflective practice is the critical component in this learning experience as it allows us to access what worked well and what did not, and to learn from our own mistakes and successes. In other words, it allows us to use theory and develop our practice in a real-world setting.

In this way, translating our reflections into action is crucial to our development as health and social care professionals. However, the reflection is only useful if it informs, develops and changes our practice for the better.

Reflection and critical reflection

Some theorists make the distinction between reflection and critical reflection. The difference is usually related to depth and breadth. Reflection can just be about ourselves and some relatively straightforward analysis of what we have done and how, or it can be a very in-depth look at ourselves and our attitudes and assumptions. It can involve a critique of the wider context in which we practice and a questioning of some of the professional processes we may take for granted. In some ways, this can be viewed as a continuum and students starting off on the road to becoming a reflective practitioner may begin at one end and progress through to being a critical reflector as they become more confident in their self-awareness and their knowledge of the health and social care context within which they are practising.

How do we do it?

We all probably reflect in an informal way all the time in that we look back over things that have happened, re-play them and wonder about why they happened as they did. Sometimes we talk things through with a friend to get their opinion or just to have someone listen to our story. Reflective practice is just a more formal and more analytical way of doing this and inasmuch as it involves writing something down, it captures something that we can then use over and over again. If we merely talk it through we may well forget some important points in what we said and decided: life as a student on placement and as a busy health and social care professional does not allow much time to stop and muse. Writing things down gives us a lasting record of our learning and learning processes, which we can then use in supervision or write up for our portfolios as evidence of our learning.

Exercise 1

This is a piece of writing just for yourself – no-one else need ever read it.

Give yourself 15 minutes; find somewhere quiet where you will not be disturbed. Think back over your week. Think back to getting up in the mornings. Can you remember one day when you got up and everything went really well? Where you got where you needed to be without having to rush?

Recall that morning. What happened? Try to write down everything you can remember about it from the moment of waking up?

- (?) Who else was there?
- (?) What did you do?
- (?) What did they do?
- (?) What happened?
- (?) How did you feel?
- (?) What else was going on?
- (?) What is the strongest memory from that morning?

Now re-read what you have written. What can you learn/take from this that might make a difference to future mornings? Can you identify the positive factors that made your morning go well? How can you make sure you have them in place more often?

Reflective practice is not just about learning from our mistakes it is also about identifying what works well, what our strengths are and how we can use them and capitalize on them in different situations.

Reflective partners

Reflection need not be a solitary pastime. Many theorists advocate having a reflective partner. This should be someone known to you who you can trust and with whom you can discuss your reflections on a regular basis. It will work best if it is someone who will ask you questions you have not thought of and put things to you in a different way. In doing this, they can open up another angle on what happened and why and may be able to offer you new insights into your practice and your learning.

Issues of confidentiality must be considered if you are discussing service users with anyone else. You may want to draw up a formal contract when you decide to work with a partner, one that delineates the boundaries and focus of your work together.

Exercise 2: Choosing a reflective partner

Think about how far you want to be challenged. Is the person you are thinking of working with someone who you think will reinforce your own views of things, or someone who may be able to challenge you in a good way and edge you into the realm of critical reflective practice?

(?) What do you have in common with this person?

(?) What is different about you both?

(?) What sort of person might you find it more difficult to work with and why? List some attributes.

(?) What sort of person would you most naturally work with? List some attributes.

(?) Does the person you are thinking of working with have attributes from both lists?

Writing up your reflections: some tips

To get started, you need to feel motivated and clear about what you are setting out to do.

➡ Set aside time each day and each week. Make it a priority.

➡ Buy yourself a writing book to become your reflective journal. Try to find one with a lovely cover that you like looking at and a new pen, again, one that you particularly like.

➡ This journal will be your log, containing the descriptions and thoughts about what you have been doing and feeling, which will form the raw material for your more structured reflections.

➡ Write in this book every night after placement

➡ It does not matter what you write or how you write it – you can even draw in it if it helps you capture a thought or feeling!

➡ Give yourself permission to write anything you want about your day, from capturing the tiniest feeling to writing about a very significant event – it does not matter.

➡ **Always be aware that you should maintain confidentiality at all times. Whether you are writing about a service user or a placement educator you should not use real names or any details which could identify them. Make sure that your journal is kept in a safe place that other people cannot access.**
➡ **Amuse yourself, write a poem, a story or write up another view of what happened. Try writing the incident from the perspective of the service user or your mentor or supervisor. See what happens, allow yourself to experiment and use your imagination.**

This journal is not for anyone else but you. It is yours to do whatever you want with and the aim is for you to access your thoughts and feelings about your practice experiences.

These are very personal journals and you will find your own style. If they are to be useful to you, you will probably need to experiment until you find a way of recording your experiences that allows you to express your own individual experience of your practice.

Use this journal as the basis for more structured reflections. Below is an extract from a fictional reflection diary kept by student nurse H. Read through it and we will see how nurse H develops it later into a critical incident reflection and then draws out what he has learnt about what happened.

Example 1: excerpt from H's reflective journal

Really busy morning on ward. Awful. Rush, rush, rush. Getting everything and everyone ready for ward round and MDT. No time to talk to patients. Three staff off sick – one agency nurse on. D in bad mood. ☺Consultant late in the end and we had half an hour sitting around waiting, trying to do things but not wanting to start anything that was too important in case we had to drop everything when the big chief consultant arrived. Alright for the others – they went back to their offices and I had to ring them when he appeared. I feel like I'm running around after everyone else and not being able to do what I want to, which is spend time with patients. I sometimes feel like everything revolves around the doctors and no-one notices us – no wonder so many people are off sick. No-one seemed that interested in anything I said either when we did eventually have the MDT. By lunchtime I was shattered. I hate the way this place just saps my energy. I'm just a little ant in this place, scurrying around in the grass, not able to see above the tall blades of grass at what is going on – but having to keep my ear to the ground to be on the look out all the time, to listen for the thud of approaching danger. I feel lost, no-one else near me that I can talk to, not sure what I am supposed to be doing and where I'm supposed to be going. I wish I could find my group and they would help me.

The above extract is an example of someone describing a busy ward round morning on a ward where the student nurse felt very uncomfortable for a lot of reasons. He ends the piece with a seemingly trivial section about feeling like an ant but this extract reveals much more about, for example, how he sees and feels himself to be so small and lost in the huge set-up of a busy acute hospital. It conveys a *quality* about his feelings rather than any more facts about what happened. It is this quality of feeling that he can then pick up when he uses this extract later for a more structured reflection.

Later on in this chapter we will see how nurse H uses this little entry from his journal to expand into a critical incident reflection where he can identify what the issues were for him, what contributed to those issues and what he needs to do about them so that he can develop his practice. He goes beneath the surface of what happened and draws out the analysis. The journal entry and the way he has written it allows him to re-engage with the feelings and events of that morning.

Critical incidents

These are often referred to in the reflective practice literature and students can often think that 'critical' means negative but it does not. Try to think of 'critical' as meaning' significant', so that it refers to anything that sticks in your mind for whatever reason when you think back to a day or a week. Some students find it easier to think about 'gut feelings', when something really affects them and they can tell this from the way they physically feel about it, for instance, a knot in the stomach or a warm glow. It does not matter whether it is positive or negative, it is significant in some probably as yet unknown way.

There are many formats for writing up and analysing critical incidents but they usually follow the pattern below to include describing what happened, exploring feelings, weighing up or evaluating what the issues were, analysing key factors, identifying further learning needs and planning what you need to do in the light of this.

Description

This is simply a description of what happened and it helps to put as much detail in here as you possibly can. Although you may think some details are irrelevant, sometimes it is only when you start to analyse things that you realize the significance of what appeared to be trivial details. You never know what will turn out to be important. Your descriptive skills will improve the more you do this, so do not be discouraged if you find this difficult at first. You can use your senses as a prompt. When describing the incident or event, think about any smells, sounds, taste, sights, etc. Describe the people who were present, the setting you were in. Nothing is irrelevant.

Feelings

In this section you can think about what you were feeling at the time but also any other emotions that were expressed by others. So ask yourself how you felt at the time, before the event, during and after. What was going on with you? How do you think other people felt? Could you tell from their reactions? What emotions were expressed throughout the event – anger? sadness? elation? joy? irritation?

Evaluation

In this section you need to start making some judgements about how the event went and what happened that was significant. Ask yourself, how do you feel the event went? What went well and what could have gone better? Try to put as much detail in here and do not just concentrate on the main thing that went wrong or the main way in which it went well. Even if you are reflecting on something that you felt went really badly, it is very likely that within that situation some things went according to plan or even really well!

Analysis

In this section you need to try to draw out the key factors and influences and what they mean. You need to look at the event in two ways, both from a personal point of view and a professional point of view. Putting everything together, the theory and policy with what happened in your case, what was it that made this event go well or badly? What happened that you did not expect to happen? How does what happened relate to any other of your experiences? What or whose intervention made the most difference and why? You need to include the wider issues here and that may include ethics, values and codes of conduct, professional boundaries and responsibilities. How did they affect the situation and how you felt about it? What is at the heart of this event for you?

Making sense of it all

Following on from this analysis and what you think was at the heart of the situation, what do you feel you have learnt from this and what would you do differently next time if this situation were to happen again? What would you do more of? What would you do less of? What do you need to explore more? What do you need to find out more about?

Action planning

How are you going to make sure that you get to where you want to be? How are you going to make sure you move your learning on and develop your practice? What do you need in terms of learning resources expertise or feedback?

This type of critical incident review can form the basis of your discussions in clinical supervision. It can provide evidence of your reflective skills and, by getting you to identify specifically personal learning needs, it can help you to really utilize the personal learning contract to its fullest (see Chapter 4 on writing learning objectives).

We will now look again at the morning's events described previously by nurse H and see how he develops them into a critical incident reflection.

Example 2: Excerpt from critical incident review from student nurse H

What happened?

Thursday morning was ward round and MDT so the morning handover was shorter than usual. D, my mentor and ward manager, took charge of the handover. She appeared to be quite irritable – she didn't drink the tea I had made her and she kept interrupting staff when they were talking. It wasn't like her. She looked tired. Three staff rang in sick and one of the agency staff from the night agreed to stay on – although I could see that D was not happy with this. I tried to take in everything they said at handover – I think it's really important to know what sort of night people have had, and I was quite worried about Mrs G in bay 2 as she wasn't well at all yesterday when I went off duty. The consultant, Mr F, was supposed to be arriving at 9am so we really had to get going getting everyone fed and washed and the meds done. I hate having to hurry people but there were two support staff down so it was all hands on deck this morning. I dashed through the jobs, hardly had time to even talk to most of the patients – D kept coming to see what I was doing – I felt like she was checking up on me. It was just gone 9am when I got back to the nurses station. All the others were standing around – the physios, OTs and social worker, all chatting. D was on the phone so I showed them in to the room where we were going to meet – only to have D follow me in and tell me that Mr F's secretary had just phoned to say he was going to be late – she couldn't say how long but it could be an hour or so – so D sent everyone out and told them I would ring them when he got here. They went away moaning – as if it was my fault! I asked D if I should go and check on Mrs G and check her radiography appt had been arranged – she snapped back at me that she shouldn't have to tell me what to do. I just stood and stared at her – then went and saw to Mrs F. I'd been with her for a few minutes and she was starting to tell me about how ill her husband had been and she was quite upset when I heard D calling me. The consultant had arrived after all and D wanted me to let the others know. I was really fed up now. I called them all and they wandered back up. The ward round was uneventful and the MDT afterwards a waste of time – the consultant didn't seem to listen to anyone else – when I started to tell them about Mrs F's husband he dismissed it and told D to follow it up if necessary. I went away for lunch that day feeling the most negative I have ever felt about nursing. I wondered if I could hack it after all.

Feelings

I felt as though no-one was listening to me, that I had no right to make any demands because we were all so busy. I felt so unimportant – like I was bottom of the heap. D is supposed to be my mentor but she had no time for me at all – and we all had no time for the patients so I felt really frustrated. There was obviously a lot of irritation about – D was like that before the meeting even got delayed – but everyone seemed to be like it by the time we got to the meeting. D looked very stressed and tired.

Evaluation

The meeting did not go well from my point of view because everyone was annoyed with the way we all had to hang around and wait for the consultant. I had to walk away from an important interaction with a patient just because of the consultant's position in the hierarchy of the team – his time is more important than any of ours. Because of the need to be ready for this ward round and the fact that we were short-staffed, the patients had a bad morning too. It can't be very nice to be rushed like that and not have the time to talk to people – particularly when some of them are in pain. Thinking of the positives, it was good to talk to Mrs F though and she obviously trusts me to be able to open up to me like that – and I actually got loads done in that first hour – I quite surprised myself how efficient I can be when I try. I didn't react when D 'told me off' either – so I'm learning to keep calm!

It was a very busy morning, with a short-staffed ward and a tight deadline which was then moved. We should have been able to cope with that – and we did – I just did not like the way it made me feel and the way it interrupted what I wanted to do in terms of good practice.

Analysis

A lot of it was to do with my feelings about the hierarchical nature of our medical teams where one person's skills and time are valued as more important than others – our professional traditions are changing but there is still quite some way to go. If I think about myself – I was resentful of the other members of the MDT, swanning back to their offices, they didn't seem to be busy yet there we were run off our feet. The staffing levels on the ward are kept at such a minimum that any absences cause problems – ten years ago this level of staffing would have been unacceptable.

Management v professional duties – it was important to get the meeting and ward round going on time – but so is personal care for the patients – we need to balance these somehow.

We all have off days – it was obvious D was feeling stressed when she arrived. No-one asked her how she was, was she ok – is that another hierarchy thing?

Conclusions and learning

I feel that team working is at the heart of this – knowing where we fit in to the team (me) and respecting each others role within it (me and everyone else) and related to that – communication – making sure that we all communicate what is going on for us, what we expect of each other within the confines of a busy, short-staffed acute ward. Things are always not going to plan – it's so complex and so many people have to come in and out of the picture – we need to be flexible to that and it has to work both ways. It would not have mattered if I was five minutes late getting to the MDT meeting – I could have carried on my important talk with Mrs F and then joined the meeting. If that had happened I would have felt better, more professional, and Mrs F (hopefully) would have felt better, better cared for and listened to. I can discuss this with D and I can work on my own assertiveness and communication skills. She would normally listen to me and if she thought I was right she would agree – even though she appeared to be tired that day – I should have tried to explain my position.

I don't feel as a student nurse I can discuss how D is feeling, but maybe as a team we could talk more or acknowledge more about how we all are. I know there is *research on team working and best practice* – I can find that out and maybe use it at one of the development meetings and identify it as one of my learning objectives to look at team processes and communication.

Action plan:

In supervision

➡ ask for feedback from D about my assertiveness and communication skills
➡ clarify expectations around student role and levels of autonomy

➡ discuss ward round/MDT and flexibility.

Next week

➡ organize to spend time with physio, OT and social worker to learn more about their roles
➡ lit search on team processes in nursing and health care teams.

Models of reflection

There are many models that have been developed to provide a structure for this type of reflection. Essentially, these models are prompts to our thinking. They can help to ensure that we are going through the whole process of reflection and in enough depth to enable us to find new insights on our practice, which we can apply and use in the future. They can provide a clear focus for our thoughts and analysis. They can enable us to develop from reflectors to critical reflectors, to question and challenge ourselves and our practice in ways in which we may never have thought of.

The main types of models tend to be one of two structures – circular or lists! The *circular type models* have been developed from Kolb's learning cycle (1984) and Gibbs (1988). They ask you to describe, analyse and action plan from an event and the circular framework encourages you to see it as an ongoing process – so that what you have learnt from analysing your practice or learning in this way is directly fed back in to what you do next time.

List type models, like the one created by Boud, Keogh and Walker (1985) and Christopher Johns (2004), are a way of making you ask yourself some in-depth questions about what happened in a developmental way – from the event, from you, to the wider context and deeper professional and personal learning.

Exercise 3

Read these models, try them and find one that suits you best. Think back over your week and find something that happened that you still feel is unresolved in some way; perhaps it is something that you feel a bit ambivalent about. Try writing up the event in the three different ways: one completely unstructured where you write whatever you like; one using a circular model; and one using a list type model. Which do you think you get the most from and why? What does each model tell you that the others do not? What does that tell you about your reflective style?

Now it is up to you. Try the journal, try the models, just start putting pen to paper! Your educator or mentor will be assessing you in many ways. One of the ways will be through direct observation of your practice but they will also want to know that you are a self-directed learner with the ability to develop your practice and your insight into your own learning. By developing your reflective skills, in the way described previously, you can demonstrate to your educator or mentor that you are doing just this.

Chapter outcomes

Having read this chapter you should now:

➡ have a greater understanding of the role of reflection in your learning
➡ have formats for recording your reflections
➡ have some idea of the models available to assist you in developing a critical reflective style.

References and further reading

Boud, D. Keogh, R. and Walker, D. (1985) *Reflection: turning experience into learning.* London: Kogan Page.

Gibbs, G. (1988) *Learning by Doing. A Guide to Teaching and Learning Methods.* Further Education Unit, Oxford Polytechnic.

Johns, C. (2004) *Becoming a reflective practitioner.* Oxford: Blackwell.

Kolb, D. (1984) Experiental Learning: experience as a source of learning and development. Prentice Hall.

Rolfe, G. Freshwater, D. and Jasper, M. (2001) *Critical reflection for nursing and the helping professions: a users guide.* Basingstoke: Palgrave.

4 Writing learning objectives

- **What are learning objectives?**
- **Writing your own learning objectives**
- **Evaluating your objectives**
- **Applying this to your placement**
- **Learning objectives levels**
- **Writing learning objectives**

By the end of this chapter you will be able to:

➡ understand learning objectives for your placements
➡ identify the overall learning objectives for your placements
➡ establish your initial learning objectives for your next placement
➡ review and rewrite your learning objectives as required
➡ transfer your learning to other learning objectives on your course.

This chapter will provide you with the opportunity to really explore learning objectives. If you can crack the code of understanding and writing your own learning objectives there will be many positive benefits for you during the rest of your course. In the world we live in today many things have to be identified by the use of learning objectives, such as service delivery, personal professional development in annual reviews, etc. Initially you may find learning objectives a little daunting to write, especially if you have never been required to write them before but if you persevere it will be well worth the initial investment.

Everything that you do at university is divided into modules including placement. Each module has its own learning objectives. Remember that coming to university is like going to another country with a different language, culture and traditions. Initially it seems strange but before long you have embraced different aspects of the things you found difficult at first, you may even come to enjoy some things as you develop personally and professionally throughout the duration of your course.

There are many debates about the interchange of the terms 'learning outcomes' and 'learning objectives'. Have a look at your course documentation. What are they called in here? For the purpose of this chapter we will use learning objectives as the terminology, to describe what you hope to achieve on placement.

What are learning objectives?

Learning objectives help to clarify for you and your educator what the purpose of your experience is in that particular practice area. Alongside your assessment form, they can enable your individual needs and developments to be clearly identified. What is your reason for being there? You are probably thinking, 'Well, to learn, obviously!' Learning objectives are the nuts and bolts of that learning and enable you gradually to learn more deeply as you develop throughout the course. There is so much to learn and you cannot possibly do it all on one placement.

Learning objectives can create clear boundaries and expectations for all parties, and provide a medium for negotiation. There are three groups of learning objectives: first, those of your own professional body, Nursing Medical Council or the Health Professions Council; second, those of the placement; and, third, the learning objectives that you set for yourself.

During placement you have to be assessed as competent to practice at the level that you have reached at the current time. This means that if you are a first year student you will be expected to perform at that level and not at the same level as your educator. Learning objectives can help to individualize your assessment both in terms of your own personal and professional development and within the practice area, so you need to use them to your own advantage! They are also invaluable if you are struggling on placement. They can highlight to your educator and yourself areas that you are struggling with and areas that you are developing.

Writing your own learning objectives

Let us start by having a go at writing your learning objectives for an aspect of your course. First, do not panic! Initially you can write them in your own language and, hopefully, as you work through this chapter you will be able to refine and revise them until it becomes second nature to think in this way. Take a couple of minutes to think about the next challenging thing that you are going to do on your course. What would you like to achieve when you have completed it? Write this, in your own words, in box 4.1. We will come back to this at the end of the chapter.

Box 4.1 Learning objectives

1.

2.

3

4.

5.

As an example, our learning objectives for this chapter would be:

➡ By the end of this chapter you will be able to rewrite the above statements in learning objectives which are appropriate to your level of learning.

Moving on

You may have heard the acronym S.M.A.R.T. to describe how to write learning objectives, we will explore this and then you can go back to your original objectives and evaluate them. Evaluation is just a word to suggest that you look at what is good about your objectives and what is not so good, so that you can improve and develop.

S.M.A.R.T. stands for:

S – Specific
M – Measurable
A – Achievable
R – Realistic
T – Timed

Go back to the objectives you have written about the next challenge on your course (we will come to placement objectives later). Have a look at each one and give yourself marks out of ten in terms of it being a SMART objective, using the chart below.

Award yourself the following marks:

⇒ Two points if it is *specific*, this means that the meaning is exact, explicit, precise, detailed, and is certainly not in any way vague. Be honest about your self-assessment, it is a fantastic skill to have, and much easier to criticize yourself than to hear it from other people.

⇒ Two points if it is *measurable*, can you demonstrate that you have done it? If so how? For example, if you can rewrite all your learning objectives at the right level we could clearly see if we had achieved our objective or not.

⇒ Two points if it is *achievable*, for example, being able to perform initial assessments on your first placement on the first day would be seen as unrealistic and therefore unachievable. It would also demonstrate your lack of insight and expectation of the situation.

⇒ Two points if your objective is *realistic*, managing the interprofessional team during a year two placement?

⇒ Putting things like, 'answer the phone' at year three is also not really realistic as you would be underachieving if this was an objective at this level.

⇒ Two points if your objective is *timed*, this needs to be clear, by the time you have finished working through this chapter, how much time have you set for yourself, in the next hour, day, week, fortnight.

If you are struggling with this, why not look at Chapter 7 on time management and then come back to this chapter.

Evaluating your objectives

Write in how you could try to improve your objectives in box 4.2, this will help you to analyse your own performance objectively.

Well done. Sometimes it can be difficult to analyse and criticize your own work, but it is an essential skill that you will need, as that is exactly what you will be doing every day as a health care professional for the rest of your career. Critically analysing and evaluating your own work is the bedrock of your continuing personal and professional development. You can use it as evidence to maintain your licence to practice. Remember we talked about the objectives validated by your own professional body? It may be useful to look these up and read them if you have not yet done so. It is also far better that you critically evaluate your own work yourself than to have someone else do it for you!

Applying this to your placement

Hopefully, now you will have some understanding of what learning objectives are. You will need to begin to apply this to your placement. This is hardest when it is your first placement and you do not know what the area is like that you are going into. If this is the case for you, then you will need to study your assessment form. If you have been on placement before, then you will have completed one assessment form (or possibly more) which will have identified your strengths and areas for development, if this is the case you can start reflecting and then identifying some clear objectives.

Check out Chapter 3 on reflection if this is a difficult area for you.

Box 4.2. Evaluating your objectives

Objective	Specific	Measurable	Achievable	Realistic	Timed
1.					
2.					
3.					
4.					
5.					

Box 4.3 Assessment forms

Identify the **main** areas that are being assessed from your assessment form.

1.

2.

3.

4.

5.

The main areas on your assessment form normally fall into similar categories whichever course you are undertaking in health and social care. The categories are usually processes that underpin your practice, such as your communication skills, your own personal and professional development or the working practices in your area, policies and procedures, health and safety, etc.

Take each area that is identified on your assessment form (box 4.3) and write an objective in the box below (box 4.4), (no more than five are required initially).

When you go on placement you will want to present as a person that has reflected on their strengths and needs, a person that has put some time and effort into planning and preparing for placement. Reviewing these objectives with your educator is something that you can discuss on your pre-placement visit or you can put it on your agenda for your first supervision session. Once you have reviewed these initial objectives together, you will be able to expand and write more objectives that are relevant to your placement learning and the expectations of your educator. You will also be able to review them at the halfway point and re-evaluate your performance. If you are not on placement at the moment you can get together with other students or ask your tutor to look at them with you.

Box 4.4 Initial placement objectives

1.

2.

3.

4.

5.

Have you checked that your objectives are SMART? Evaluate them against the criteria you used earlier and give yourself marks out of ten. Try to make sure that you have got a range of objectives that are a balance of things that you think you do well at and things that you would like to develop, and that cover the main areas that you are being assessed on.

When you discuss these objectives during your supervision session it will hopefully enable you to remain focused on what you have to achieve to pass the placement, and will also provide you with evidence of what you are going to do, how you are going to do it and when you are doing it. The objectives will only do this if they are written SMARTly. In other words if they are:

Specific
Measurable
Achievable
Realistic
Timed

You will be able to increase your ability to write, rewrite and evaluate your objectives the more that you discuss and reflect on them during your placement and during supervision. There are many packs in universities explaining how to write learning objectives, maybe you could check out your learning against some of them.

Learning objectives levels

Now that you are a little clearer about writing learning objectives, we need to discuss levels. We will refer to first, second and third year, if you are on a part-time route or other pre-registration route you will need to adjust this slightly and be clear about the level of placement rather than your actual year.

As well as being SMART your objectives also need to be at the right level for your stage of learning, remember you are not expected to be at the same level as your educator at the end of the placement. You do need to be aware of the theory that you have learnt up to this point within the university and begin to integrate this into your placement learning.

In a very small nut shell at the first year, you are explaining *what* you are doing. For example, that you will meet the patient, carry out an initial assessment, identify the person's needs, identify the communication skills you need to be aware of, and so on. You should begin to use models of reflection to help with your personal and professional development and identify your strengths and areas for development.

At the second year you should be furthering your reflective skills and answering the questions you should be constantly asking yourself when on placement. For example, 'What am I doing?' or 'Why am I doing X?' or 'How am I going to do Y?' This should enable you to explain to anyone the *what, why and how* of what you are doing. For example, why are you carrying out an initial assessment and how are you going to carry out the assessment? Think about things like your verbal and non-verbal skills, your observation of the client's communication, what information you need to gain from the service users and most importantly at this level, *why*. This will include things that you may have covered in university like evidence-based practice, professional reasoning, etc. They are also chapters covered in this book if you need to revisit them.

In your final year you will be doing all of the above and also asking yourself questions such as: 'Was that the best way to do X?' and 'Could there be a better way?' and 'How does it fit in with the latest government initiative/trust strategy/departmental policies and procedures?' and 'How can I find out about it and change my practice?' Your reflective skills should be used throughout, and it goes without saying that this final placement should be the culmination of all of your learning on previous placements and at the university.

If you are still not sure, take some time and write more objectives and evaluate them using your assessment form as a guide to help you. Ask your personal tutor to evaluate them with you and give you feedback.

Have a look at the objectives in box 4.5 and try to evaluate them. Decide which ones are well written and why, and which are poorly written and why. Write your comments in the right-hand column.

Box 4.5 Sample learning objectives

Learning objective	Your comments
Year 1	
1. Understand the dynamics of the team.	
2. Describe the assessment process in this clinical area to the team.	
3. Identify the main health and safety factors to be aware of when working with this client group.	
Year 2	
1. Select, carry out and evaluate an appropriate assessment for the patient.	
2. Develop my communication skills.	
3. Analyse and justify using professional reasoning, the selection of a treatment intervention for a service user.	
Year 3	
1. Independently carry out an assessment, critically analyse and suggest alternatives supported with evidence.	
2.Critically evaluate my own performance after my first independent intervention using an identified reflective model.	
3. Describe the discharge procedure.	

Hopefully things are starting to slot into place. Have a look at our suggestions and see if you have said the same.

Year 1	Your comments
1. Understand the dynamics of the team.	
'Understand' is too vague, think of your behaviour and how will it change when you understand what you will be able to do?	
'Describe and explain using a diagram the team dynamics' would be better.	
2. Describe the assessment process in this placement area to the team.	
This is much clearer and states how you are going to explain either verbally or using a presentation what the assessment process is in this placement area.	
Year 2	
2. Develop my communication skills.	
'Develop' is again too vague. What will you have to do to develop them and how will your behaviour have changed as a result of your development?	
Maybe you could write and analyse verbal and non-verbal communication during an assessment using a reflective model and identify specific areas to work on. You could review this in supervision and receive some feedback on this.	
Year 3	
2. Critically evaluate my own performance after my first independent treatment inter-vention using an identified reflective model.	
We could examine this learning objective to see if it is S.M.A.R.T.	
Specific – You have taken responsibility for your own learning and have identified how you will do that.	
Measurable – You will have a baseline of your initial performance and will be able to compare this formative performance to your summative one and use this as evidence in supervision of your development.	

Year 3 cont.	Your comments
Achievable – It appears achievable if you identify time for reflection after your session and for feedback during that week's supervision session.	
Realistic – It is a realistic expectation for someone at your level to want identify their strengths and areas for development, to self-monitor and to provide evidence of personal and professional development.	
Timed – You have identified when you will complete the critical evaluation.	
3. Describe the discharge procedure.	
You should be doing more than describing in your final year. Instead, you should be critically evaluating the discharge procedure, for example, saying what is good about the discharge procedure and what is not so good. You should always be supporting this with national and international research, suggesting alternatives and, as in year 2, illustrating how it fits in with national and local strategies and procedures.	

When we started this chapter we asked you to write in your own words learning objectives for an aspect of your cause and then we have been working through the process of polishing these objectives using 'university speak'. This time we would like to see if you can work the other way around. We will give you the describing word for a year and you can write what you think it will mean in your own words. This translation, although strange, is something that you will come to be familiar with during your placement.

On placement two languages can be used: *medical language* and *lay language*. Lay language is the common language, sometimes referred to as slang, but it is the language used by the person in the street. In your professional capacity you will need to speak both medical language and lay language, as you need to be able to speak both to people who have no clinical knowledge *and* to experts in the specialized field. For instance, a client may refer to having had a 'bit of a funny turn', which can be described as lay language. The consultant may confirm that the person has had a T.I.A., Transient Ischemic Attack, which is the medical term.

The same principle applies to academic language. As we have just explored, your practice tutor may ask you to analyse an assessment tool. You may need to think about what is good about the assessment and what is not so good then you will need to find articles and relevant research to support your statements. For example, you may use phrases such as:

'This person says Y, however, this author suggests Z about this kind of assessment. Alternative assessment tools are … They also have strengths which are … and limitations which are … On balance it would appear that this assessment tool is a valid tool to use in this situation because … And my evidence to support this is …'

If you are still struggling with objectives and language, console yourself that you are doing exceptionally well considering that you are trying to get to grips with two new languages, academic and medical, simultaneously.

In box 4.6 below we have listed some of the common descriptors used in each year of your study, starting with Year 1 and moving through to Year 3. Try to identify exactly what you think each word means in the context of your practice placement, starting from your own level. Write this explanation in your own words, and then the knowledge, skills and attitude you need to demonstrate your application of this on placement. We have filled in Year 1 to get you started.

Box 4.6

Year 1	Definitions/explanation
Explain	Tell the educator that an assessment was used to gain information about the patient/service user.
Comprehension	Understand why that information was required and how it was used.
Identify	Recognize the assessments that were used in this placement area.
Describe	Observe my supervisor carrying out the assessment and feedback the verbal and non-verbal communication skills that they used during the assessment.
Discuss	Read and become familiar with the assessment before talking about my ability to carry out an assessment with a patient.
Year 2	
Illustrate	
Analyse	
Compare and contrast	

Year 2 cont.	Definitions/explanation
Examine	
Plan	
Year 3	
Critically analyse	
Critically evaluate	
Judge	
Construct	
Teach	
Create	

Well done. It is not easy but you have made a great start. Try to use the academic words as much as possible and then like anything they will become second nature.

Writing learning objectives

Now you should feel able to go back to your original learning objectives and rewrite them as SMART objectives. Before you start the next chapter, try writing some learning objectives for yourself.

Now you can focus on your placement and write learning objectives which will be SMART and clearly identify what you wish to work on during your next placement. This will be a great start to the placement and provide evidence of your reflection, insight and ability to self-assess.

Chapter outcomes

Now that you have completed this chapter you should feel more confident to:

➡ describe what learning objectives are
➡ identify the level that you are currently at
➡ write some learning objectives for the next chapter
➡ write at least four learning objectives for your next placement
➡ critically analyse these and revise them.

Well done you have completed this chapter.

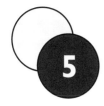

5 Assessment

- **Introduction**
- **Preparation tips**
- **Preparing for placement assessment**
- **The pressures of being assessed**
- **Being assessed**
- **Assessment – playing your part**
- **Preparing for self-assessment**
- **Making good use of time**
- **Keeping motivated during placements**
- **When things become difficult**
- **Formative assessment**
- **Halfway through**
- **The summative assessment**
- **The assessment process**

By the end of this chapter you will be able to:

➡ understand the components of assessments on your placement
➡ identify the minimum standards of competency required at each year of your training
➡ be clear about the terminology of assessment – formative and summative
➡ be able to self-assess competently and confidently.

Introduction

This chapter will provide you with an opportunity to explore what is being assessed during your placement and how the expectations of your knowledge, skills and behaviour will change as you progress through the course and each placement.

All the other chapters of this book should come together here and you should be able to identify where your strengths are and what areas you need to develop in a broad perspective in relation to your placement. Most assessment forms are developed from the competencies required of a health and social care professional in their first job. These will obviously be specific to your own profession. The competencies are broken down further so that they link with the academic development of your course, starting with 'describing' at first year and working through to 'critical evaluation' at third year. Placement development should be reflected in how your learning objectives change as you work through the years. It is unlikely that you will be asked to do anything on placement that does not contribute to your development as a health and social care professional.

The thought of a continual assessment can feel quite daunting before each placement but you must remain focused on your goal which is to demonstrate competence at your level of placement. Competence has many different definitions but basically you will be expected to demonstrate the skills, knowledge, attitudes, understanding and experience required to perform in professional and occupational roles to meet the minimum standard of your year of training. So no-one is expecting you to have the knowledge and skills of a state registered professional on your first placement. A common anxiety among all students is the thought that they have to be as good as their educator by the end of the placement. This is simply not true. Take a good look at your current assessment form and the minimum standards required to pass at your level. This will enable you to break the requirements down into objectives and demonstrate your achievement of these by the end of your placement.

Remember that because competence is the demonstration of your knowledge, skills, behaviour and so on, you can do some preparation before you go on placement.

Preparation tips

➡ Examine your assessment form for your next placement and make sure that you read it thoroughly.
➡ Identify any areas that seem unclear. These are the areas that you really need to clarify and understand *before* you go on a placement.
➡ Set yourself a date when you can sit down and work through the assessment form. You could do this in pairs or a small group.
➡ Maybe you will work through the assessment as part of a university preparation session. If not, as you go through the course there should be other members of the group who have had experience in different placement areas and maybe able to help out with examples from their own experiences. Beware, though, every placement is different so treat this information just as a guideline.

Some preparation for placement is well worth the investment and will give you the best possible start on placement, even if you do not know which placement area you are going to. Working through the assessment form will give you a basic understanding of the expectation and level of practice required.

Preparing for placement assessment

Let us look at some things that you can do to familiarize yourself with the assessment form and think through some of the things that you will be able to do during the first couple of days, or week, on placement to familiarize yourself with the department. (This can be done even before you know the placement area you are going to.) Go back to the main areas that you identified from your assessment form. They probably included some of the areas we have identified below. If not, use a photocopy of your assessment form.

Here are some ideas to get you started, although obviously you can adjust them to your year of training:

Assessments

❶ Identify the assessments used in this area.
❷ Read through the assessment and make sure I understand what it is asking.
❸ Observe my educator carrying out the assessment.

Communication with other professionals

❶ Make a list of the people on the team.
❷ Arrange visits by the end of week one.

This should give you an initial idea of things you can do, but see if you can fill in some more areas from the main areas on your assessment form. You may want to rewrite some of these when you find out where you are going on placement, but most should apply to all placements, and you will be able to adapt them as you go through the course and become more experienced. Review how you are assessed, for example is it pass/fail or are you graded on a scale 1–5 or A–F? Make sure you are clear about the expectations of the different grades that you are expected to demonstrate at a pass level and what would be required from you to receive an excellent 5 or A grade on the assessment form. Make sure you do this early enough in the placement to allow you to incorporate the requirements into your objectives and then provide clear evidence of how you have achieved them.

The pressures of being assessed

Box 5.1

Jot down some of your anxieties about being assessed.

Sometimes placement assessment can feel like climbing over a never-ending mountain range. Those thoughts and feelings that you have about assessment can also be used productively as they can give you empathy with the clients/service users that you are working with. Some of your feelings about being assessed are exactly the same as your patients/clients or service users have when you are assessing them.

Some of your thoughts and worries might have included the following:

Will I do it right?

What if I make a mistake?

How will I know if I have done anything wrong?

Will anyone tell me?

What if I fail?

Are these similar to the things that you have thought about? Maybe you can add to the list above with other things that you have thought of.

Do not forget about the patient/client here. Do you give them the same opportunities to explore their anxieties about the assessment? Do they know why they are being assessed and what the assessment will be used for? Remember how it feels to be a patient or client, and that *you* have chosen to be there in your professional capacity.

Being assessed

Throughout the placement you will be being assessed in many different forms depending on the nature of your placement. Initially, before you are 'let loose' on the general public, your educator will provide you with the opportunity to observe them in action on the placement. Then, when either you feel confident or your educator feels it is time for you to carry out an intervention, you may do it together or you will be observed completing the set task. Don't worry, you are not expected to be perfect or do it to the standard that you have observed. Remember that you are learning and your educator is already qualified. Everyone knows how difficult it is to be observed as everyone will have been observed at some point in their professional career. Educators are aware of how it feels to be observed and how that alters the dynamics of the situation. Your educator is responsible for you throughout the placement and they need to feel confident that you can cover the basics and that you will refer back to them if you are unsure of anything. Your educator will also rely on feedback from other members of the interprofessional team, any person you arrange to visit and also service users. Most placements will also expect you to present information to the rest of the team either in meetings or at a formal presentation at some point during your placement. This should only be a consolidation of your learning on the placement. Each week in supervision you will be able to receive feedback about how the assessment is progressing and whether you are meeting the minimum standards required and demonstrating that you are competent to practice at your current level. This is why your learning objectives should link in with your assessment form.

Box 5.2 The assessment form

Make a note of the main areas of assessment on your assessment form.

Hopefully, you will have some of the following on your list:

➡ Professional communication.
➡ Personal and professional development.
➡ Working practices.
➡ Assessment, treatment intervention.

Often these main 'umbrella areas' are broken down into component parts. You should become really familiar with your assessment form before you go on a placement then you know exactly what is expected of you. You can explore areas that you do not understand or areas where you are not sure what is expected of you in your preparation sessions at university or on your initial visit to the placement area. You will feel more convinced of your abilities if you have a very clear idea about the knowledge, behaviour, skills and attitudes that are expected of you on the placement. If you can, have a copy of your assessment form with you as you are working through this chapter and then you can continually refer to it and become more familiar and confident with it. Look at the minimum standards that you have to achieve to pass your next placement.

Assessment – playing your part

When you go on a placement it is equally as important as it is at university to play your part and take responsibility for your own learning. Make things easier for yourself by ensuring you carry out a pre-placement visit, so that you know where you have to go on the first day, how to get there on public transport or where to park, etc. You will also then have a rough idea of the time it takes to get there. Visiting the department will also provide you with an opportunity to meet the educator before you start and maybe other members of the team. You will be able to observe the dress code and ask about tea/coffee breaks, lunch, start and finish times. You will also get a 'feel' for the place. If you send a CV before you go, your educator will be able to plan for you. There is nothing worse than the student who arrives on the first day and has had no contact with the area. Your educator will have no knowledge about you or your previous experience. Instead of beginning the placement in a positive light you begin the placement in a negative one and will spend valuable time trying to turn around the image the educator has about you. If, however, they have met you and read your CV, they may be able to plan visits/groups/clients that would build on your existing experiences.

Do not worry, though, if the placement has only been finalized at the eleventh hour, which is common, as this obviously does not apply to you, but be prepared and have your CV at the ready.

It cannot be said enough times that you must prepare for the placement and remember that you have to achieve the minimum standards of the assessment form by the end of the placement and not on day one.

While you are reading the next section, think about any anxieties you may have about a placement. Running through events in your mind and visualizing yourself in the situation can sometimes help to reduce anxieties. Remember that the vast majority of students love being on placement as at confirms with them why they are on the course – so think positive!

Preparing for self-assessment

Imagine you are on placement now. Ask yourself about the highlighted words on your assessment form: do you feel comfortable and understand how you can prepare yourself, even before you know where you are going on placement? Are you clear about your role? Rate yourself out of ten for each of the key areas identified in box 5.3 as a way of self-assessing what areas you need to focus on. All the areas highlighted in the list are chapters in this book, so all you need to do is make a note of the areas where you do not rate yourself so highly and then review and work through the relevant chapter.

Box 5.3: Self-assessment

Take a brief look at the chart below and, in the spirit of self-assessment, give yourself a mark out of ten to demonstrate how confident you feel about each area.

Subject	Marks out of ten	Date identified to work through the chapter
Preparing yourself for placement		
Balance and time management		
Reflective practice		
Writing, learning outcomes		
Portfolios and progress files		
Supervision		
Interprofessional perspectives		
Complex decision-making and professional reasoning		
Failure		
Evidence-based practice		
Integrating university and placement learning		

Looking at the chart above, what are you doing well at and what areas do you still need to work on? Go back to the chart and look at any areas that you marked yourself as less than five. These are the areas that you really need to read around and understand *before* you go on placement. Set yourself a date when you can sit down and work through the relevant chapter(s). This will give you the best possible start on placement, even if you do not know which placement area you are going to, as working through the chapters will give you the basics that are applicable to every situation. Remember that by completing this chapter you have already demonstrated that you can self-assess!

You will find a chapter on all of the areas outlined above, so you can keep going back and reviewing where you are up to and how you are developing with each skill. You should have made a note of the dates from your initial self-assessment and allocated some time to read around the areas you have rated as less than five. You may also want to allocate some time to re-read all of the chapters before you go on placement, if you have not gone out on placement already.

Above all, as you work through this book and go on placement it is important that you be honest, realistic, try to keep motivated and focused, and that you ask for help when you need it, and, hopefully, you will pass all your placements with flying colours. If you do experience any problems we have included a chapter on failure, which will help you understand some of the reasons why placements sometimes fail.

If there are any outstanding issues you should discuss these with your university tutor or educator when you are allocated one. You will have the following opportunities to assess yourself and get feedback as you go through your placement(s):

➡ You should be having weekly supervision in which you can ask for feedback on your progress on the assessment form.
➡ You will be reflecting on what you do so that you can offer your own self-assessment of the situation.
➡ You will be writing and revising your learning objectives in conjunction with the assessment form and your educator.
➡ You will be developing your professional reasoning which will demonstrate your understanding of what you are doing and why.
➡ You will be able to arrange visits with other members of staff to demonstrate, among other things, your ability to manage your time, your understanding of the roles of other professionals and your communication skills.

Making good use of time

When you are on placement, especially in the earlier part of the placement, you will have time when your educator is busy on the phone or in discussion with others, or off sick, or in a meeting and so on. If there is nothing specific for you to do you may feel at a loose end. You will feel more purposeful, and indeed will appear more professional, if you have a number of small tasks that you can be 'getting on with'. All the things that you have now identified can be carried out in the first couple of weeks and will add to your formative assessment.

Keeping motivated during placements

Box 5.4: Keeping motivated

Write down the five main reasons why you wanted to come into this profession.

   1.
   2
   3.
   4.
   5.

Keep the thought in your mind that this is the profession that you have chosen and in order to do it well you have to:

➡ learn and demonstrate to others that you can do your job competently and safely
➡ understand why you are doing what are you doing (what the evidence base is)
➡ understand what the reasoning is behind your decisions (professional reasoning).

The practice placement assessment will enable your educator and the university to consider if you have met the minimum standards of competency identified by your profession and university at your current level and whether you are able to continue to the next level of your training and eventually become state registered. The state registration is an assurance to the public that you are safe to practice, and that you are continually keeping up-to-date and can provide evidence that you are competent to practice.

If you are struggling to come up with five reasons why you entered the profession then you may find placements difficult. You need to talk things through with your university liaison tutor, as the motivation to receive state registration and become a professional is the main thing that drives the majority of people through the course and the placements. If you are unsure about your motivation to be a professional it could be one of the reasons that you are a bit half-hearted with your interest in the assessment form, or maybe you are just exhausted from a night shift at a residential home, or night out, in which case get some sleep and come back to this later!

As we have authorized, your state registration and place on your professional register demonstrates to the public that you are safe and competent to practice. Your practice assessments at each level at university are the rungs on the ladder to reach your state registration. Focusing on your goals can help if a placement is difficult. Think about where you would like to work eventually, and what you can gain from this placement that will help you on that journey. Even if you are not enjoying the placement and it is not an area in which you would like to work, it is crucial for your development and you need to pass it!

When things become difficult

When you are on a placement that you are not enjoying or finding difficult, remember you need to pass the assessment to achieve your goal, try to think how you can turn the things that you are finding difficult to your advantage in terms of your own career development. Use Chapter 3 on reflective practice to try to understand yourself a little better – a vital skill when working with people.

Let us have a look at some of the reasons why you might be finding placement difficult or you feel that you are not enjoying it, and what you can do to turn the situation to your advantage. If you are not enjoying a placement you can withdraw from the placement but usually this will count as a failed placement and the implications are that you will have to resit the placement at another time, reducing your holiday and possibly putting you under extra pressure and stress. Initially, you will have to reflect on the situation. Is it just that you have a bad feeling about the placement itself, but actually during supervision your educator does not indicate that anything is wrong? This could be the best scenario as you are actually passing the placement and your educator has not indicated that there are any causes for concern on your assessment form.

Has your educator had feedback from another member of the team or do they feel that there are communication issues? Some of the things that initially appear problematic can be used to your advantage and also provide evidence of your development on the assessment form. Below we work through some of the most common issues that students face on placement and suggest some ways forward and potential solutions.

Not getting on with your educator or member of a team.

If you are in this situation and are not getting on with someone in your team, be it your educator/mentor or someone else, then we would suggest that you reflect on the incident or explore with your educator how you are coming across to others, and why they feel there are problems with your communication. What are the observable behaviours that you have demonstrated?

Ask yourself some questions:

 Has this been fed back to you before?

 Are you aware of the behaviour that you are demonstrating?

 Are you tired or working while on placement?

 Do you want to change the behaviour?

After you have explored all these questions and tried to find some answers, go back at the next supervision session and discuss this with your educator, indicating that you would like to change your behaviour. The reality is that *you* have to pass the placement not your educator, but do not forget to feed all the information back as soon as possible to your university liaison tutor if you are unhappy.

During the next supervision session you can then identify an objective for your assessment form that you can work on during the week and receive feedback.

A possible suggestion could be, 'To actively work to communicate with all members of staff and explore their roles during a selected point during the patient journey.'

This approach can make it easier to keep the emotion out of the assessment, it will keep you focused and will provide evidence for the educator of a range of your skills including your commitment, motivation, communication skills, and your understanding of interprofessional working during the patient journey.

Formative assessment

Your formative assessment will normally be carried out about halfway through the placement and as the word suggests it is a shaping and determining assessment. It will clearly feedback to you how you are doing, what is going well and which areas you still need to work on. Hopefully, you will have been reflecting throughout the placement and have self-assessed by this point so you should have few surprises.

Is important to listen to the formative assessment and not become too defensive. Take the assessment away and think about it. Think about the following:

 How closely does it link to what you were already thinking?

 Does it roughly say the same things as your own self-assessment?

 Is it a million miles away from your own assessment? In which case, it is time to discuss things with your university liaison tutor.

Halfway through

Once you are settled into the placement you will know the routine: the assessments, the record keeping, the different interventions, etc. You will have received your halfway report and have reflected on it. You will have revised your learning objectives too, but it is important that you do not become complacent because at this point the placement is not over. Bear the following in mind:

➡ Be clear about your revised objectives. Make sure that they are at the right level for your stage in training and reflect the feedback you have been given.
➡ Have a good look at the assessment form. Go through all the components, how can you demonstrate that you are competent? Is that reflected in your learning objectives?
➡ You should have a better understanding about your educator.

What makes them tick? What makes their blood boil? If things have not gelled together then do not worry, you have made it this far. Keep objective, keep focused on the assessment form and demonstrate what you can do.

The summative assessment

Again as the name suggests this assessment sums up your overall performance on placement. It is your final assessment from the collective total of all that you have achieved on this placement. Once more, you should have been able to assess yourself before your educator has assessed you and, hopefully, there should not be any surprises if you have had regular supervision and feedback throughout the placement.

If you have not had regular supervision or feedback and there are surprises, then you may wish to feed this back to the university. If you have actually failed, remember that while it is horrible and feels like the end of the world, it is not. If you are in this situation, then start by reading Chapter 12 in this book on failure. Then talk to everyone who will listen, go through the rest of the chapters again, be critical of yourself and generally reassess where you are personally and profession-ally. Then, arrange a meeting with your university tutor and decide which options are open to you.

Often during the summative assessment it is tempting to switch off as you have completed the placement and know that you have passed. Interestingly, this is the time to listen most closely to the feedback that you will receive. On balance, most educators write positive things about students in the final report. The verbal feedback which supports this can be the most revealing and should be noted. If all is well do not worry about the report as long as you can understand everything that is written and the rationale to support it. Your educator is relaxed now their role is almost over and they can go back to normal. Listen and take discrete notes about the things that they say about you that are not written down, for example, any anecdotes, how you first came across in the department, what surprised them about you, and maybe even what drove them mad about you initially. You can learn a great deal about yourself if you are open and listening to that feedback, and it is feedback that you can use on the next placement or as you go forward to a career.

The assessment process

Once you have completed an assessment you can heave a sigh of relief, the placement is over and you have passed ... phew! However, the assessment process is not over. In fact, we are sorry to say that it never really ends. As a health and social care professional working with people you need to continually review your work, judge yourself, evaluate and consider the work to be done and completed. Working through this placement you have not only demonstrated that you have the knowledge and skills required to progress to the next level, you have also demonstrated an understanding of assessment at its many levels:

➡ assessment of yourself
➡ assessment of a client/patient/service user
➡ assessment of a service.

Now that you are at the end of this chapter, think about something that you have learnt about yourself while working through this chapter. It can be anything, however small.

This has been a tough chapter, so congratulations for persevering through the activities. We hope it has helped you in your understanding of assessment.

Chapter outcomes

Now that you have completed this chapter you should feel more confident to:

➡ understand the components of your placement assessment
➡ identify the minimum standards of competency required at each level of your training
➡ be clear about the terminology of assessment – formative and summative
➡ be able to self-assess competently and confidently.

Well done, you have completed this chapter.

Further reading

Alsop, A. and Ryan, S. (2001) *Making the most of fieldwork education: a practical approach.* 2nd edn. Cheltenham: Nelson Thornes Ltd.

Neary, M. (2000) *Teaching, assessing and evaluation for clinical competence: a practical guide for practitioners and teachers.* Cheltenham: Stanley Thornes.

Stuart, C. (2003) *Assessment, supervision and support in clinical practice: a guide for nurses and other health professionals.* Edinburgh: Churchill Livingstone.

6 Complex decision-making and professional reasoning

- **What is clinical reasoning?**
- **The service, the service user and you as the professional**
- **Definitions and categories of professional reasoning**
- **Chapter outcomes**

By the end of this chapter you will be able to:

➡ identify the factors involved in complex decision-making
➡ analyse the reasoning processes involved in practice
➡ identify the links between your learning needs, the needs of the service users and those of the service itself.

As a student in the practice setting you will be faced with making complex decisions on a daily basis. Talking to service users, answering their questions, deciding on how to proceed with their case, discussions in team meetings, reflecting on where to go with your input with a service user – all such decisions are based on your professional reasoning skills. This is about more than just your professional knowledge and skills, it is about how you use that knowledge and those skills in the specific context of your placement.

Working with people is not a science, it is an art. There is never one solution that will be the answer to everyone's problems. Even if you work in a highly specialist service where you only see people who have very specific needs, there is never one solution that will suit everyone. You may have a standard approach or model that you work with, but you have to apply it on an individual basis with every single person that you see.

In order to make our practice appropriate to every individual we deal with, we need to draw on a range of knowledge, from our professional knowledge base, to our emotional intelligence, to our knowledge of the service we are in.

Professional reasoning can involve just one decision you make with a service user, or it may be integral to the whole on-going input you have with someone. It is a process rather than a skill. It is the articulation of the thought processes behind the decisions we make together with the service users on a day-to-day and long-term basis. It is our justification for those decisions and can be tracked and developed as we learn more and more about ourselves and our professional abilities.

What is clinical reasoning?

Clinical or professional reasoning involves using your professional judgement, and is based on: your specialist knowledge; the service user's individual needs and priorities; their emotional state and personal characteristics; ethical principles and the boundaries or restrictions to the service you can practically provide. It is a process of balancing the needs of the service user with your knowledge and skills alongside the remit and boundaries of the service you are placed in. It is a process that is ever changing and evolving as the situation and needs change day by day or even minute by minute. It requires you to be able to adjust and change your input with a service user as the situation demands, basing your judgement on a synthesis of knowledge from all the above aspects.

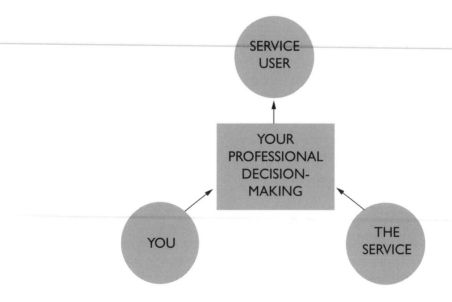

Figure 6.1 The components in decision-making

Example 1

You are a social work student working with a family who have drug and alcohol problems. Your role is to encourage them to access support services for their young children and to keep them together as a family. After two long sessions with the parents, together you decide on a package of support for the next six weeks. You have discussed this at length with your practice teacher and have agreed a plan of action. The next week you visit to find that the father has left the home and the area, the mother is distraught and drinking heavily. You realize you may need to re-think what the priorities are and alter the support package totally. With the service user you will have to weigh up the priorities and statutory obligations, your knowledge of what other support services there are, and together decide on a new way forward: professional reasoning in action. You would then go back and check this out with your educator again.

As a student on placement, you are not expected to be an expert from day one, people learn to be experts. Your placement is a *learning* opportunity and each experience you gain will allow you to develop that expertise as you discuss issues in supervision and reflect on your learning. This is not just a one-way relationship either: you always have something to give to the service you are learning in. Your honesty and experience – based observations should be welcomed by your service. You are in a unique position as a student who comes into an established service. You may be able to see things from another point of view or from a different angle, one that the permanent workers in a service may miss because they can become overfamiliar with the routine of day-to-day working. A forward-thinking, developing service will always listen your opinion.

When you are involved in the process of making decisions with service users about their needs you may be aware that from time to time you are out of your depth. It is important that you are able to identify this. It may be that you do not have the theoretical knowledge. Perhaps the person has a medical problem you have never come across before. Perhaps they want a service you know little about. Perhaps you feel you are unable to cope with the emotional upset the person is expressing. When you feel like this it is a sign to consult your educator. The service user knows you are a student. If you (clearly, but very respectfully) tell them that you may need to talk to your educator about what they have been discussing, they should be reassured. There may be cases where you do not tell the service user this explicitly if you feel it may damage their confidence in you, but you may still be able to do this after the interview with the service user is over. You should always check complex decisions or unusual choices with your educator, but do not necessarily rule them out.

Let us look at this complex relationship between you, the service user and their needs and the service of which you are a part.

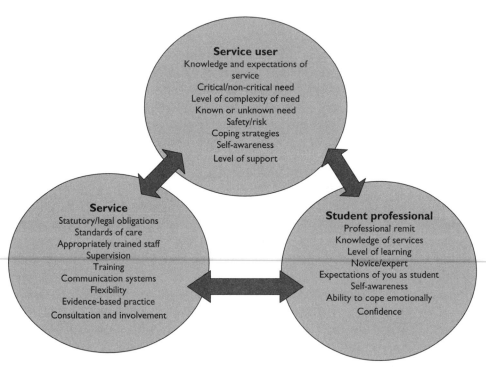

Figure 6.2 The relationship between you, the service user and the service

The service, the service user and you as the professional

The service in which you are working has statutory and legal obligations to provide certain services within certain boundaries and at certain standards of care. For example, accident and emergency services are set up to provide an immediate assessment and treatment service for people experiencing trauma. They are not there to treat on-going chronic or minor conditions on a day-to-day basis. They have certain guidelines as to the time within which a person should be seen; they have certain standards of care as to what should happen to patients, the types and numbers of trained staff and the skill mix of those staff, the types of assessment patients can expect to receive according to the trauma and the types of treatment they can expect to receive. Accident and emergency services will have relationships with other parts of the service; for example, wards that can be accessed if needed and other parts of the health service which relate to their service, such as GPs and mental health services. All these aspects are set down in the trust regulations for that service. In addition, the service user wanting to access this service has certain needs. These needs are:

➡ knowledge of what that service is there for and what is available
➡ knowledge of how the service works and interrelates with other parts of the service
➡ expectations about how they will be treated and by whom.

The student on placement in the service needs to know:

➡ what their service can provide
➡ what their professional role is in it
➡ what is their remit as a student
➡ what other services are related to it.

Definitions and categories of professional reasoning

Definitions of the different types of reasoning vary from theorist to theorist. Below are some of the most commonly agreed forms of reasoning. Do not become bogged down in the definitions, as they can often make something more complicated than it is. What is discussed is a thinking process, something that you will do as a student on placement all the time with everyone that you meet and in every case you work with. It is useful to list them for you to reflect on your own practice in each placement you go on:

❓ Which types of reasoning do you tend to use more naturally?

❓ Are there some types of reasoning that you do not feel as confident in using as others?

❓ Are there certain types that you have not considered before?

Do some practice settings lend themselves more to one type of reasoning than another?

Procedural reasoning

This refers to the body of knowledge and skills that come from your professional knowledge base and it is sometimes also called scientific reasoning.

Example

Your knowledge of musculoskeletal problems and the effective treatment for specific injuries as a physiotherapist, or your knowledge of the law and child protection procedures as a social worker. When faced with a person with a particular need you know where to start. You would not advise a person with a cartilage injury to try soaking the limb in hot water, for instance. You would know what to start thinking about in terms of treatment. Obviously, this knowledge base grows the more experienced you are but there are specific expectations of you at each level on placement. Certainly by the time you qualify in your chosen health and social care profession you will be at a required, agreed level of knowledge.

Questions to ask yourself to help your procedural reasoning

 What do I know about the symptoms and prognosis of this condition? or What do I know about the legal requirements in this situation and the services needed to support this person?

 Have I ever seen someone in this situation before? What are the similarities and differences?

 What do I *not* know about this situation and where can I find out about it?

Conditional reasoning:

This refers to the context within which the service user lives their life and how that impacts on your suggested treatment or approach with them.

Example

You are a physiotherapy student working in an orthopaedic outpatients clinic. You are treating a young man after a severe tibia and fibia fracture following a road traffic accident. You are aiming to build up his muscles following wastage after external fixation. He attends every week but shows no sign of having followed his exercises at home in between sessions. You read in his notes that he has had to move back in with his parents since the accident and that he had previously been in shared accommodation with friends. When talking to him about this he says that his parents are very protective of him and tend to do everything for him with a result that he is feeling very demotivated. You consult with your educator and suggest that you bring him in to the unit three times a week for a while and for him to join an exercise class run on the unit. This would bring him back into contact with other young people and may motivate him to take control of his recovery again.

Questions to ask yourself to help your conditional reasoning

(?) What do I know about this person's life? Where they live, who they live with? What job they do? How they spend their time?

(?) How does this effect the treatment I might suggest?

(?) Will they be able to carry out the treatment I suggest given their lifestyle?

Narrative reasoning

This refers to the part that narrative plays in all our lives and influences how we react to something. As a student professional in health and social care you will be dealing with people who are in some kind of difficulty or after something traumatic has happened to them. In order to give the person the most effective input that you can, you need to understand not only what has happened but what this *means* to them. Narratives are about how we construct meaning in our lives, they are how we make sense of our lives and they are our stories about ourselves.

By listening to someone's story of what has happened to them you can begin to see what it means to them and how they see their life. If they have been through a traumatic event then what they thought was going to be their future, where their story was going (or their predictive narrative), may well have been shattered and they may now face a different future than the one they imagined.

Example

You are a community rehabilitation nurse. The person you go to see has had a stroke at 65, two years after retiring. The person was looking forward to many years of active retirement. They had joined lots of local groups and were a busy part of the local community. The stroke has left them unable to walk and with minimal use of their left arm. They now face a different future to that which they were expecting. It is your role as a professional in health and social care to negotiate this changed future with the person. If you understand what their original narrative was for themselves you will understand more of what they must be going through. If you understand to some extent what the person is going through, then your treatment and interaction with them is likely to be more effective in the long run. Part of what you will be doing with this person is creating a new narrative of the future. This will be one which is acceptable to them, not one which is just about what you think should be done for a person after a stroke.

Questions to ask yourself to help your narrative reasoning

What does this illness/problem/situation mean to this person and their life?

How do they see it?

How has it changed their view of themselves?

How will they cope with a new future?

Interactive reasoning

This refers to the way that we, as professionals, pick up on emotional signs from the service user about how they feel about what we are saying or suggesting, and use this information accordingly, to engage them in treatment or change our suggestions.

Example

You are a student nurse on a mental health placement. You are working one-to-one with a woman who is experiencing an episode of debilitating anxiety. There is an anxiety management group running at a local resource centre and you think this would be a useful service for them to access. When you are talking to her about it you notice that she seems more anxious. You pick up on that and check out with her that she would feel alright about attending it. She says she would go but her body language leads you to question whether she is just saying what she thinks you want to hear. You suggest that you attend with her for the first session and she visibly relaxes a little. She begins to open up about her fears of appearing foolish in public and becomes more talkative. You have taken heed of the non-verbal signals between the two of you and used the interaction to inform your decision-making with the service user.

Questions to ask yourself to help with your interactive reasoning

Have I really listened to everything the person was trying to tell me – including thinking about their non-verbal communication?

How do they seem when I am talking to them about what we are going to do?

Have I the skills to deal with their feelings? If not, can I talk this through with my clinical educator/mentor?

Pragmatic reasoning

This refers to the boundaries surrounding what you can offer people. These boundaries can be financial, geographical or involve time limits. You can rarely do all you would like because services have regulations and limitations. You do not help anyone if you promise things you cannot deliver, but at the same time it is quite a skill to be able to work around these barriers and find alternative solutions to issues.

Example

You are a community occupational therapist in a service for people with learning disabilities. You have been working with a family around the best position and seating for their son with severe cerebral palsy. The family are very isolated and this is impacting on the mother who is the main carer. She has friends and relatives in nearby towns but is becoming depressed by her isolation. You have been working on the seating for the house for their son but you are aware that he needs a very specialist type of chair that is not readily available and beyond their means to purchase. You have thought around ways of compensating for this, which is as much as you can do at the moment, and you know your department budget will not condone more expense. You do not give up, however. You research grants available from charitable bodies and find one specifically for disabled people in isolated rural communities. You apply and receive funding for a specialist chair which can be used in the house or car. This enables the family to go out together and the mother to take her son out and for her to keep up the social contact she needs to be able to cope.

Questions to ask yourself to help with your pragmatic reasoning

Am I aware of the limitations to the service in terms of what we can offer – financially, geographically time wise?

Have I been clear with the service user about this?

Have I thought of possible ways around these barriers if necessary – looked for alternatives? Who can I ask about these?

On placements in health and social care settings, you will be dealing with complex decision-making on a daily basis. In making these decisions and using your practice educator or mentor for support, you will find yourself using all the above professional reasoning styles rather than just one style. One way you can develop your learning and your confidence is to analyse your reasoning and see how you are considering the range of issues around the service and service user to give them the best possible outcome.

Below are two examples of students using all these styles of professional reasoning skills as part of their everyday work.

Example 1

You are a second year nurse on a placement in a GP surgery. You are taking a drop-in clinic for women with your nurse mentor. This is the third time you have done it together and she is happy for you to see women on their own in the room next to hers. She pops in between patients to talk to you about how you are doing. You have taken a routine blood pressure (BP) check for a new self-referral. The woman's BP is way above normal and when you tell her the results she becomes very upset and tells you that her life is very stressful at the moment. She confides in you that she is in serious debt, her job is very insecure and she has taken on a second job in the evenings to try to pay off some of her debts. Her best friend has recently left the area and she feels completely isolated and lonely. She is not sleeping well and is comfort eating and putting on weight. She says she feels out of control of her life and does not know what to do.

(?) Where would you go from here?

(?) What can you do in this setting?

(?) How would you respond to this woman?

Using your clinical reasoning skills you would look at the problem from many angles.

❶ The central issue that you have uncovered is her high BP. As a nurse in a GP surgery you would need to make absolutely sure that you dealt with this and how you go about this would be crucial. There would be a professional protocol for this. This demonstrates *procedural reasoning*.

❷ How long do you have to talk to this woman? Are you confined by appointment times? Do you have time to go further into the problems she is bringing up? If not, what can you do in the limited time you have with her to show her that you have listened and heard what she said and is there any advice or help you can point her towards? This demonstrates *pragmatic reasoning* – you may be very limited by the small amount of time you have to give this person, so what can you do that will be most beneficial in this amount of time?

❸ What support does she have around her? What is her day-to-day situation like? Does she have any flexibility at all in her life where she could maybe take some time out from work? Are there any ready-made support systems in her life that you could encourage? This demonstrates *conditional reasoning*.

Example 2

You are an occupational therapy student on placement in a community mental health team for older people. You have done your first initial assessment on a woman who has moderate dementia. Mrs B lives with her husband and they are supported by the community team as and when they need it. Mr B is asking for advice and help to engage his wife with something to do during the day as she is spending a lot of time just sitting and appears to becoming low in mood.

You arrive with the details of her cognitive assessment and her activities checklist, which lists her hobbies, so you have a fair idea of the types of activities that she may be able to engage in with some support (*procedural reasoning*). Your task is to marry up what she may be able to do, with what is possible in the environment, what she is motivated to do and what her husband can help her with (*conditional reasoning*).

However, when you start talking to her about what she would like to do, she becomes very upset and talks about losing everything and being useless, and being treated like a child. You change tack and when you talk to her about her life (*interactive reasoning*) she identifies that her home and garden were her pride and joy and it seems to you that her whole sense of self came from doing those two aspects of domestic work and she visibly brightens up and becomes more animated when she is telling you about this (*narrative reasoning*).

You bring the husband into the conversation more and it appears that he is now doing all the domestic tasks and the garden as he thought this was helping his wife. In discussions that follow, all three of you look at how Mrs B could be more involved in the day-to-day tasks, with Mr B's support, and you offer to explore the possibility of support from Home Care to facilitate this.

You take this back to your practice educator and look at the risks involved and the resource implications for Home Care (*pragmatic reasoning*).

The above examples illustrate the range of components and processes involved in your day-to-day decision-making in practice. You use a variety of resources, view points and judgements to make these decisions with the service user. You do not need to be able to identify what you are doing as you do it, but analysing your decision-making process like this brings these things to the surface and allows you to make that process explicit. In this way you can develop your practice skills as you become more familiar with the ways of looking at things and applying your theoretical knowledge to the specific situation you are faced with.

Having read this chapter you should now:

➡ have a framework which can help you think through your decisions
➡ have an understanding about the different needs of the service user, you as a
learner and those of the service in which you are placed.

Further reading

Higgs, J. and Jones, M. (2000) *Clinical reasoning in the health professions.* Butterworth-Heinemann.

Johnson, B. and Webber, P. (2004) *An introduction to theory and reasoning in nursing.* 2nd edn. Lippincott Williams.

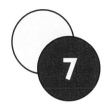

7 Balance and time management

- **Introduction**
- **Where are you now?**
- **Reasons for the imbalance**
- **Developing realistic time frames**
- **Prioritize your tasks**
- **How can you put your decisions into practice?**

By the end of this chapter you will be able to:

➡ identify your work/life balance
➡ make decisions about where you are and where you would like to be
➡ prioritize your tasks and allocate a realistic time frame for these to be completed
➡ explore the reasons for your work/life balance
➡ decide how you are going to put these decisions into place on your placement.

Introduction

This chapter will provide you with an opportunity to examine your time management and organizational skills. You may be tempted, because of your limited time, to rush through this chapter and not carry out the exercises and just read the conclusion. However, that would be a complete waste of your time! This is your life, so give yourself some time to examine it, and if you need to put some strategies in place to change the way you feel. It would be time wisely invested.

Becoming a health and social care professional does not happen over night and requires some self-reflection and personal development on the journey, as well as writing assignments and being on placement. The first step on that road would be to identify an hour in which you can explore some of the issues, and examine your time management and organizational skills using this chapter.

If you cannot identify an hour in which you can do this, you need to stop right now! You *need* to read this chapter and adopt some of the skills and approaches it will teach you, otherwise you will be burnt out before the journey has begun!

In exploring your work/life balance, you need to look at your life. It may be useful to picture your life as a circle with all your roles and responsibilities as segments within it. Think about your life for a moment, by the day, week and month. Maybe it changes all the time but overall you feel balanced. Maybe you consistently feel that the balance is not right, and that you would like to do something about it.

If you think this, maybe you would like to invest an hour of your time in this chapter. You may reap big rewards in terms of your health and well-being. This will impact on your placement. You will appear calmer and be able to give your attention to your placement area knowing that you are doing the best that you can in difficult circumstances. Even if you think you are organized at university, when you go on placement it can throw up a whole host of other issues as you try to juggle travelling, study time, organizing visits, carrying out assessments to name but a few things.

Box 7.1 Identify your work/life balance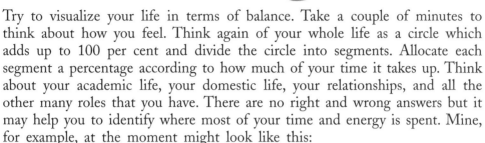

Try to visualize your life in terms of balance. Take a couple of minutes to think about how you feel. Think again of your whole life as a circle which adds up to 100 per cent and divide the circle into segments. Allocate each segment a percentage according to how much of your time it takes up. Think about your academic life, your domestic life, your relationships, and all the other many roles that you have. There are no right and wrong answers but it may help you to identify where most of your time and energy is spent. Mine, for example, at the moment might look like this:

➡ Mother 65%
➡ Wife 15%
➡ Daughter 5%
➡ Sister 2%
➡ Academic 10%
➡ Friend 2%
➡ Time for self 1%

Now do your own:

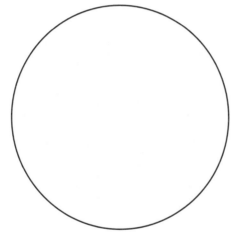

Great, you are one step closer to achieving more balance in your life. We will come back to this at the end of the chapter.

Have a look at your circle. Does anything jump out at you? Is there anything which surprises you? Anything that you are unhappy with? If all the segments are exactly as you would wish them to be and you are happy with them, then well done, you have already got balance in your life. If they are not you will need to reflect on this. What is dominant and why? Where would you like to make changes? Do not worry if you think it is not possible as even a small shift can make an enormous difference to how you feel and can make you feel more in control of your life. If you can identify and prioritize your roles, you may feel a little calmer and more in control, and identify possible shifts for where you allocated your time while you are on placement.

Where are you now?

Stop for a moment and think exactly what you have to do, in the next hour, day, week, by the end of placement. Balance and time management inextricably link your personal life with placement. So it is likely that you are thinking about tasks you need to do, such as food shopping, chores or washing clothes, alongside thinking about writing, learning objectives and arranging a visit, or reading up on the placement area. Use you own sheet of paper if you need to break this down further or you have more things to add. Use the table on the next page to work out what you have to do in the immediate and less immediate future.

Box 7.2

In the next hour	By the end of the day	By the end of the week	By the end of the placement
Example: Complete chapter on balance and time management			

You should feel a little better getting all those thoughts down on paper, or perhaps they look even more overwhelming!

The next stage is that you need to try to identify roughly how long each task will take, remembering that using words like 'forever' will not do. If you feel that this is the case then you need to be more pragmatic. Why not try breaking down what you have to do into smaller pieces, which is great practice as part of your life-long learning as a health and social care professional. Once you have given it some thought, write your honest estimation of the hours it will take you to complete each task. We will return to this chart later.

Reasons for the imbalance

There are many reasons why your life can feel unbalanced. Some of them might be due to good reasons like the start of a new course or relationship, while some might be not so good, such as due to a sudden illness either of someone close to you or yourself. It might simply be an assignment deadline or planning a group or assessment on placement, which is making you feel this way. Often going on placement will involve a change in routine, getting up at a different time, getting a different bus or taking a different route to your normal one. You will probably be out of the house for longer hours and may have to juggle childcare, relationship time, study, etc. You may even have to live away from your normal home and friends. All of these factors can have an impact.

Box 7.3

Looking back at your circle how do you think that your work and life is balancing? How will that change when you are on placement? Try to think of three main reasons why it may feel unbalanced.

1.

2.

3.

Are there any common features in your answers?

Developing realistic time frames

Having a realistic idea of the amount of time it takes to complete a task is essential to organizing your time. Applying this realism to all the tasks you have to complete between now and the end of placement is a great strength on the road to having a more balanced life. More often than not we underestimate how long it will take us to achieve things. For example, after running a group recently we estimated that it would take my co-facilitator and I, 20 minutes to debrief and write up the notes. In reality it took us an hour. That meant that to debrief and write up the notes for all of the nine sessions that we ran took us nine hours in total, when we had only allocated three hours to do it. This is six hours difference! If this is repeated with all the work and tasks you have to do at home, along with travel, planning reading for an assignment and so on, then you can see how easily it is to literally run out of time. What actually happens is that when your planning and time allocation is poor and you do not allow yourself enough time, tasks will build up and you will begin each day in time debt. This can lead to an overwhelming workload, inability to meet deadlines, stress and burnout. For this reason it is always better to overestimate the time it will take to complete a task. So if there are seven hours in your working day you will be filling that day with seven hours of work, not nine hours because your time allocation is poor. You will become aware of jobs that can fit into the seven hours and be able to prioritize them, remembering to include time to check emails, open post, liaise with colleagues, etc. This will mean that you will work more efficiently and realistically. It will mean you are able to prioritize your tasks, set realistic deadlines and make accurate predications about completing tasks as a student health care professional.

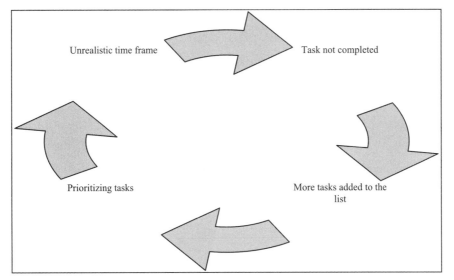

Figure 7.1 The negative effect of inadequate time allocation

Being able to identify a realistic time to complete tasks is an essential skill that you will need in your role as a health and social care professional. For example, imagine that after a case conference you have received some new referrals from your educator. You will need to identify adequately when you will be able to have an initial interview with that person, how long that will take and what else it will encompass, for example, any telephone calls, emails or liaison with other workers/carers, travelling time, writing up the notes, etc. As you can see, it includes much more than just going to speak to the person, which is the time most people set aside and why they end up in time debt.

Having the ability to think around the initial task and identify all the connecting tasks that are required will make you and the service more efficient, and will enable you to identify clearly any problems you may have in fitting it into your day or week. Remember too that it will also probably take you more time than it would your educator as often you will be carrying out the activity for the first time. For example, if as a qualified member of staff you have to create a waiting list then you will be able to provide evidence to justify this. Your code of conduct will clearly state when you must write in the notes after each session with a client, and you will have recommended standards of practice to follow for every different practice area. It may be worth exploring these before you embark on your practice placement, and while on placement make a note of all the other activities that are involved in a stated task.

Having realistic time frames will enable you to offer a quality service which includes planning and development time, which supports the service that you can offer to the client/service user.

Box 7.4

Go back to your estimations of the time that you have allocated to each task you included in the chart earlier in the chapter. Make sure that you have included all the connecting tasks associated with the activity and then fill in the chart in Box 7.5 after you have asked yourself the following questions.

Did all the tasks initially have a realistic timescale?

✔ Yes ☐ No ☐

Do you need to review and change any of the estimated times?

✔ Yes ☐ No ☐

Do you need to complete every task?

✔ Yes ☐ No ☐

Would the world fall apart if some of the tasks were not carried out until after placement?

✔ Yes ☐ No ☐

Review the tasks that you have identified for today, or tomorrow if you are reading this chapter in the evening. Identifying how long a task will take is a valuable skill to learn.

Box 7.5

Tasks	Time to complete task (hours) Including connecting activities
	Total time required:

You will not always get it right, when you do get it right make a mental note of it and you can use that information again next time. If you get it wrong then, great, you have learned something. Again, make a mental note and use that information next time.

Every time you complete a task, why not play a game with yourself such as estimating how long you think the task will take and what are the connecting tasks. How many times are you right? Often people can underestimate how long a task will take and spend their lives running around and achieving very little and acquiring hours of time debt. Two hours' time debt on Monday will become four on Tuesday, six on Wednesday, and by Friday you can have over a day's worth of work which has still not been completed. This will be added to Monday's to do list and so it continues. If you can begin to have a realistic idea about how long a task will take, based on fact, then you will be well on the way to better time management. This will impact on your personal and professional development as you progress through the course and your career as a health and social care professional.

As much as we would like time to be infinite we are aware that it is a precious commodity and one that we do not want to waste.

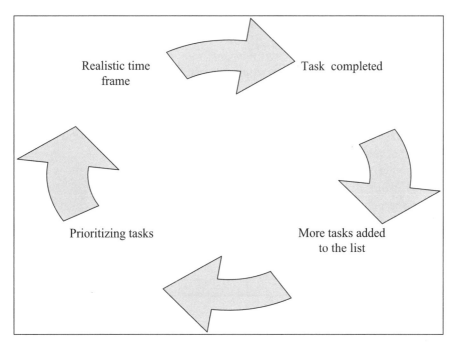

Figure 7.2 Positive effect of realistic time allocated to tasks

What does a typical morning look like for you when on placement? Your typical morning could have looked like this in your diary:

Tues 8am–12noon

Check post and emails/telephone feedback from team: 15 mins

Prepare for the group: 15 mins

Run the group: 1¹/₂ hours

New client assessment: 2 hours

When you have realistic times allocated to tasks with connected tasks your diary could look something like this:

Tuesday am 8–12 noon

- Check post and emails/telephone feedback from team.
  Connecting tasks – make coffee, talk to colleagues, reply to emails, mail and telephone review and reprioritize diary in the light of new info. Reality time taken: 1 hour.
- Prepare for the group.
  Connecting tasks – organise the room, find other chairs, find flip chart, read through notes, welcome group members. Reality time taken ¹/₂ hour.
- Run the group.
  Connecting tasks – wait till everyone has left, answer some questions from group, make coffee and check emails again, debrief with other members of the team, write up notes. Reality time taken 2¹/₂ hours.

It is easy to see that although you had agreed to carry out an assessment and run the groups, in reality you will have to reprioritise your tasks as you only have four hours in the morning and do not have any spare time to complete a new assessment on Tuesday unless you cancel the group or a colleague was able to run it for you. If your diary was set out with realistic time allocated to tasks you could easily have seen that you were not available to carry out an assessment on Tuesday morning, or you could have decided that the assessment was a priority over the group, or negotiated this with your educator.

Prioritize your tasks

Now you are able to allocate realistic times to your tasks for today (or tomorrow) it may be a good idea to prioritize them, starting in time honoured tradition with the most important task. How do you decide what your priorities really are?

Box 6

It may be useful to think about:
Which item would make you the most happiest if it was not left on your list tomorrow.
What do you *feel* that you have to do first?
What do you need to demonstrate so that you can pass the placement?

Each day you have only 24 hours. Take away seven hours for sleep and you are left with 17. Take away time spent on eating and cooking, which could be two hours; then, for example, meeting friends takes five hours. This leaves you with ten hours for everything else, and so on and so on. Do not forget about all the 'thieves' of time, such as cups of coffee, day-dreaming, rescheduling your work schedule, telephone calls, reading text messages and checking emails. The list is endless … and that is where all the time has gone, not forgetting of course family and socializing and the TV has not even been mentioned! No wonder there is so little time left to prepare for placement, read up on the area, write assignments and so on.

Box 7.7

Complete the chart below and you will be able to identify how much time you have left after you have taken away all of the activities mentioned above. This will give you an indication of how much you can realistically achieve each day. Do not forget that it needs to *balance*.

Time available each day.	Make a list of all the activities that you need to carry out tomorrow, whatever they are.	Make realistic sugges- tions of how long each task will take (do not forget connecting tasks).	Time left.
24 hours	Sleeping	7	17
17	Eating/cooking	2	15
15	Travel		
			0

Now you can focus on your practice placement, what tasks have to be completed before, during and after placement.

Box 7.8

Here are some examples, try to fit your own list into these three categories, and do not forget to add your connecting tasks.

Before placement	Realistic time frame	During placement	Realistic time frame	After placement	Estimated time
Organize pre-placement visit	1 hour phone call, write letter, update CV	Time for clinical reading		Critical reflection	
	Total		Total		Total

How can you put your decisions into practice?

Now that you are able to identify your tasks, make realistic estimations of the time it takes you to complete them, prioritize and negotiate what you can achieve each day, then you are ready for your placement. If you have your diary you can already block out time for travel and study each week. You will be able to see how much time you have left for all the other things in your life, and reorganize some of them before you start placement. If you have not got a diary, then now is the time to invest in one. It can even be a cheap blank book that you have written your own dates on, it does not have to be the biggest and best. You will need to take a diary on placement with you as you will have to book all your activities into it.

When you complete a new task on placement make a note of how long it takes and what connecting tasks are involved and how long they take. Keep a record of these times in your diary and you will be able to use this as a reference in the future.

Box 7.9

Review your diary to prepare yourself before you go on a placement. Remember placements are time limited and so some of these activities will only have to last for the duration of your placement. How much time will you have left realistically each day after travelling back from placement and preparing for the next day? What things can you do to make life easier for yourself while you are on placement? Try to write at least four things. Some examples are given below:

➡ Allocate study time in your diary.
➡ Estimate how long your day will be including travel.
➡ Identify a time to meet up with other people on your course for a drink/support.
➡ Organize food in advance.
➡
➡
➡
➡

Now you have completed the time management activities, go back to the picture of the circle on p79. How much of the segment will placement take up? What segments will have to be reduced in order to make it fit into 100 per cent.

Make a note of some of the reasons you have for altering your segments, if this is what you have done. Why you have made these decisions? It may help you as the placement progresses to come back to these reasons to keep you focused and remember how much time you have left. If you feel that there are larger issues that prevent you from fitting in placement at the moment, it maybe that you have to reflect on this and make some decisions.

Box 7.10

What do you feel is most important to you at this time in your life?

➡

➡

➡

Is it placement or are other issues more pressing? Only you know the answer, but discuss it with friends, family or your tutors. You can then make a realistic decision about whether this is the right time to go on placement, and what are the alternatives if you do not.

Whatever your decisions may be there is no doubt that, as a health and social care professional, it is your responsibility to offer a quality service to your clients or patients. Remember back to when you found out that you had got a place on your course, and how you felt about it. Sometimes the journey to state registration does feel overwhelming and daunting. If you can continue to allocate your time realistically, you will not only feel the benefits yourself but your profession will also benefit. It will enable you ultimately to identify what is a realistic service to offer in a working week, if you can work out what is a realistic time to allocate to a task or activity. Then you will be able to negotiate from a position of strength and knowledge; for example, you might need to say to your manager:

'This quality assessment will take x hours including admin, miscellaneous, liaison with others, etc. I have x hours in the day, I also need to eat, drink and go to the bathroom, so I will be able to carry out x assessments per day. To carry out any more I would need more time and/or staff or the quality of the assessments will be reduced.'

You can start this process immediately when you are on placement. Add organization and time management to your objectives, and try to write one objective now. If you find writing objectives difficult and confusing you may need to prioritize your time and identify when you can read Chapter 4 on writing objectives.

Always remember that this is part of your journey to become a health and social care professional and it is a journey that you chose. Your life can be one long round of pressure and anxiety, or it can be one in which you make choices knowing what you can realistically achieve in terms of the tasks that need completing in a day, week, or month. Being time aware gives you the platform to negotiate with other people and decide for yourself what your priorities are. This is your life and these are your choices.

Chapter outcomes

Now that you have completed this chapter you should feel more confident to:

➡ identify your work/life balance
➡ make decisions to make your life more balanced
➡ prioritize your tasks in a realistic time framework
➡ put your actions into practice before, during and after your placement
➡ provide a high quality service for your service users.

Well done, you have completed this chapter.

Further reading:

Adair, J. and Allen, M. (2003) *The concise time management and personal development.* London: Thorogood.

Clegg, B. (1999) *Instant time management.* London: Kogan Page.

8 Supervision

- **What does supervision mean to you?**
- **The nuts and bolts of supervision**
- **Preparing for supervision**
- **Reflection**
- **The supervision session**
- **Receiving feedback**
- **The supervision process**
- **Practicalities**
- **Moving on after the supervision session**
- **If things are still not going well**

By the end of this chapter you will be able to:

➡ be clear about what supervision means
➡ identify your role in supervision
➡ develop an agenda for supervision
➡ negotiate with your educator in supervision
➡ link strands of your personal and professional development to supervision.

This chapter will provide you with an opportunity to explore the what, when, why and how of supervision. Although you are free to work through the chapter whenever you feel like, you will probably get more benefit from it if you work through it just before or during your placement.

We aim to explore supervision with you and what it actually means to you and your educator. It is a dynamic concept which changes in the same way as any relationship constantly changes. Supervision dynamics can change from session to session and can even change within a session depending on the needs and expectations of each party. We explore the changing dynamics of supervision and why it occurs during your placement, and how you can play an equal role in the process. You are probably thinking, 'I just need to know what I am doing and then I can get on with it and hope to get though the placement with the least damage done to all parties.' Placement is part of a bigger picture for you and your educator.

For your educator it could be the first opportunity to practice supervision, or they could be an experienced educator who is continuing their personal and professional development by having a student. For you it is part of your professional journey and, in order to develop, you need to receive feedback on your performance to enable you to reflect and progress. Supervision is a requirement of all health and social care workers as part of the government's clinical governance framework. It enables good performance and levels of competencies to be to be acknowledged and recognized, and poor levels of performance or lack of competence to be picked up quickly and training requirements highlighted.

What does supervision mean to you?

Supervision can mean many different things to many different people, and you will already have some kind of expectation about what will happen during supervision. Jot some thoughts down about what you expect to get out of supervision. Try to write at least four things in box 8.1.

Box 8.1

* *example:* A time to talk about my case load.
*
*
*
*

Well done. It is useful to start with your expectations so that you can be clear and honest with your educator, and also you can explore your own wants and needs. The bottom line is we all want to know how good we are, and that we are not failing. Although that can be part of supervision, as you will see working through this chapter, it can give you much, much more.

Now that you have an opportunity to think about *your* expectations let us have a look at some of the expectations of your educators. These are some of the ideas that have been collected from the educators who have attended the many accreditation courses that we have run over the years.

Educator's expectations:

- Praise
- Bringing the theory and practice together
- Confidentiality
- Structure
- Trust
- Someone who is approachable
- Good communication skills
- Motivation
- Guidance
- Consolidation
- Feedback
- Assurance
- Action plans.

Make a note of how many on your list match the list of your educator's. If it is less than half then you may wish to revise your expectations of supervision!

Remember that supervision is a dynamic two-way process in that you need to be giving as well as receiving all the things you have circled on the lists. The role of your educator is to guide and monitor your performance, identify appropriate clients or patients for you to work with, as well as to negotiate the level of complexities of your learning depending upon your level of placement. They are required to challenge and support you in your personal and professional development throughout your placement.

The nuts and bolts of supervision

Now you have established what supervision is, or what you would like it to be, you need to identify when, where and how long will your supervision session be. The minimum time for supervision is normally one protected hour, once a week. Although this is stated it can often in reality be ten minutes here and 20 minutes there. It may help if you discuss supervision in your pre-placement visit, if you have one.

Supervision checklist

Do you know when your supervision will be?

✔ Yes ☐ No ☐

Do you know how long your supervision session will last?

✔ Yes ☐ No ☐

Do you know if you will be using a supervision contract?

✔ Yes ☐ No ☐

Have you negotiated who will write the agenda?

✔ Yes ☐ No ☐

Have you negotiated who will write notes from supervision?

✔ Yes ☐ No ☐

Before you start yelling, 'Yes, but last week I ...', then remember the word *normally*. There are a wide range of supervision patterns which are often linked with the placement area. You may receive informal feedback after working with a service user or in the car between visits. You should also have some formal supervision on a weekly basis. If you have not received any supervision for two weeks consecutively, or answer no to all of the above, you need to contact your university tutors. Contrary to popular belief they are not psychic, but they can help if they know there is a problem. You also need to read your placement handbook thoroughly before the pre-placement visit. Every course has different requirements for supervision. Some are pre-set and some are negotiated, so make sure you know exactly what your university course requires you to do before you even get to your placement. It may sound obvious but many people do not even know that there is a placement handbook.

Preparing for supervision

Because time is limited and supervision is precious, you need to make the most of the one-to-one time that you have to talk about yourself and your performance. If you feel there are not enough hours in the day, you may need to work through Chapter 7 on time management before you continue. You need to be objective. In order to be objective you have to review your week and prepare for your supervision session. This gives you the opportunity to demonstrate to your educator that you can reflect, are objective, can identify what you have done wrong and how you can improve. You can underpin this with your developing theoretical knowledge and, as you go through the course, your evidence-based practice and professional reasoning.

Reflection

There are many ways to unpack what has happened to you during placement and many reflective models which you can use (see Chapter 3). If you have found something that works for you then great, but if not try out this way of unpacking and analysing the layers of your thoughts and actions on placement.

The following headings will provide a straightforward way for you to think about your week and link theory and practice with your emotions. Underneath is an explanation of each heading and what it entails.

Fact and implications

What did you do? What happened as a result of what you did? This can be intentional or not.

Personal issues

How do you feel about what you have done? Honesty is the only way here.

Strategy for development

What do you need to do now?

Underpinning theory

What theoretical knowledge do you need to know to develop?

Fact and implications

You may not be aware of the implications of what you have done, for example, breach of unit policy, staff wondering why you have not returned to work after a home visit. This might be fed back to you during supervision.

Personal issues

Hopefully, you should know how you feel about something that you have done. If you do not really care or are unhappy on placement, this may be an opportunity to involve your liaison tutor from the university and explore the issues further. You may need to check out your motivations for coming on to your course, ask yourself if you would like to continue with the placement, and discuss this further in supervision.

Strategy for development

This is where your learning contract/action plan/objectives come in. How would you like to change and how can you demonstrate that you have got there? Are you working at the right level, how do you know and how can you demonstrate it?

Underpinning theory

This is the bit where you demonstrate you are able to use the learning centres, access relevant literature, provide an evidence base to support your practice, demonstrate relevant theories models and integrate them into your practice. You also have to demonstrate that you can understand theory, relate it to your practice and explain it to others. Try to work through some of the other chapters in this book and use that as evidence.

The example we have included of a student's initial interview, which you will find on the next page, illustrates the links between theory, practice and your emotions. Read through and explore it. It could help you to develop your practice in a more objective way, and take responsibility for your own change and development.

Example of reflecting on a supervision experience

Facts and implications	Personal issues	Strategies for development	Underpinning theory
Did initial interview, asked some questions I did not know the answer to. Client left with unanswered questions.	Felt like an incompetent idiot … need to do more work on reflection and analyse the incident properly.	1. Make a note of questions and find the answers from most appropriate source, discuss with educator. 2. Review history of client before next interview, try to anticipate questions.	Reflective model. Professional reasoning. Evidence-based practice.

Box 8.2

Have a go yourself, although you will probably need more paper. Think about this placement or your previous placements. If other words work better for you as headings then use them but stick to the facts, the implications of those facts for the patient, yourself, your educator, the team and service and be clear about your suggestions for improvement. And do not forget about the all important theory, placement is a fantastic opportunity to make sense of the theory as you can put it into practice straight away. You may need some help with some of the areas, but remember clarification and feedback are some of the roles of supervision and you can always add them to your agenda.

Facts and implications	Strategies for development	Personal issues	Underpinning theory

Well done, you have identified the facts, attempted to identify areas for development (this can be confirmed in the supervision session to check you are going in the right direction), linked all this to your own personal development, and identified the underpinning theory. Obviously, you will require some guidance and facilitation (this is why you are not qualified yet) to enable you to reflect, debate, examine and develop. But remember your educator does not have all the answers either!

The supervision session

From your supervision preparations try to identify the things that jump out at you. What issues are on your mind the most? What work issues do you wake up thinking about and what thoughts are still loitering in your mind when you fall asleep? These are your priorities.

What if your priorities are your personal issues?

It must be said here that, contrary to popular belief, personal issues *do* affect your placement. If you have got personal issues you will need to discuss them in supervision. To be clear, this is not an opportunity for your own therapy session, rather it is a chance to explain some of your behaviour. Discuss the facts of the situation that you are in with your educator and try to reach a conclusion. Do you need a few days off to sort things out? Or is it more serious and you feel you cannot continue with the placement at this moment in time? Whatever the outcome talk to your educator and contact the university!

Box 8.3

From your supervision prep sheet see if you can identify your priorities, things that you feel would be valuable discussion points for your supervision session. Remember you only have 60 minutes.

Agenda item	Time estimation
1.	
2.	
3.	
4.	
5.	

Do not forget your educator may have some issues to put on the agenda.

Let us just recap:

➡ you have reviewed the week and reflected on your performance
➡ you may have filled in critical incident sheets which have enabled you to identify what went well, where and how you feel you can improve, and what theory you need to understand to support your learning
➡ you may have filled in the chart in this chapter. Whichever method you have chosen you should have thoroughly unpicked and explored the highs and lows of your week.

Inextricably linked to all of the above will be your personal and professional development as you learn, reflect and develop throughout the course. You should now feel ready for your supervision session!

Receiving feedback

One of the most difficult aspects of supervision is receiving feedback. Feedback is one of the most important aspects of supervision, and receiving what you could perceive to be negative feedback can be one of the most complex issues of placement.

It may be useful to list some of the things that you may feel when you receive negative feedback from anyone. Think of a time when someone was telling you that you had done something wrong. How did you feel? Try to list some of those feelings below. This will hopefully allow you to be more objective about those feelings and help you to explore which strategies could be useful to you during supervision.

Box 8.4

1. Example: 'I just wanted to throw in the towel and say, "I can't do it." '
2.
3.
4.
5.

We are sure you could continue! We have seen things like: anxiety, despondency, generally disheartened, and comments like, 'Will I ever get it right?' These kinds of thoughts can be quite negative and subjective. Different reflective models are useful to change some of your own negative self-talk, which is often not helpful in moving you forward and can prevent you from feeling open to new learning opportunities. If you feel you could carry on with the list it may be useful to explore those feelings and where they come from before continuing with this chapter. Maybe you could try discussing them with a close friend or tutor. Self-reflection is an essential tool for a developing professional and some personal changes in behaviour and attitude would be expected at the end of the course. If you feel that you are 'stuck in your ways' or simply do not want to change, then you may find placements difficult. This will impact on your personal and professional development as you have to continually change and adapt as a student and continue to adapt and change to remain a competent practitioner throughout your professional career and maintain your state registration.

The supervision process

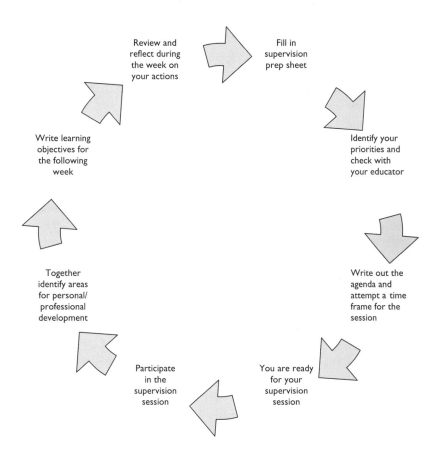

Review and reflect during the week on your actions

Fill in supervision prep sheet

Identify your priorities and check with your educator

Write learning objectives for the following week

Write out the agenda and attempt a time frame for the session

Together identify areas for personal/ professional development

Participate in the supervision session

You are ready for your supervision session

Figure 8.1 Rolling supervision process

Figure 8.1 illustrates the rolling process of supervision. It can also be used for peer supervision if one-to-one supervision is not available to you. Before every supervision session, as with everything, you will need to prepare. Think about the previous week, including what has gone well and what has not gone so well so that you try and get a balance of both. If anything stands out for you from the week, it is vital that you have the opportunity to explore and analyse it. If things have gone well then you need to clearly identify and unpack why, so that you can gain from the experience and hopefully repeat it and build your personal and professional skills. If the reverse is true and things have not gone so well, you will need to follow exactly the same process so that you *DO NOT* repeat the experience. If you do not prepare before supervision you will find that you are trying to 'think on your feet' and you can appear defensive instead of reflective and open to development. Check your agenda with your educator before supervision and add anything that they suggest. This may mean that you will have to reprioritize your own agenda so that you have enough time to discuss the issues. It is sometimes difficult to squeeze everything into a 60-minute supervision session. As you become more experienced, unpack incidents and reflect on them before supervision, and so you will be able to begin to suggest a time frame. This means both parties sticking to the agenda, which is a skill that many people try to aim for. It is good time management practice and who knows you may just about manage it by the end of the placement. You could have it as one of your objectives and that will help to keep you both focused.

Practicalities

Make sure that the room is booked and try to anticipate any interruptions; most people can wait for an hour. If you only manage 10 or 20 minutes, try to see if you can negotiate a longer session the following week. Normally your supervision will be an hour a week but be aware that this will not always be the case. Check your placement handbook as supervision is essential for your personal and professional development and if you are not receiving it, you may need to involve your liaison tutor from the university if you cannot resolve the issues with your educator. Engaging fully in the supervision session is vital as is your ability to absorb the feedback (both positive and negative) and move forward objectively to your next week. At the end of the supervision session you should both be clear about your objectives for the following week and any adjustments you have to make to your existing objectives. Check Chapter 4 on writing learning objectives if you find you struggle writing these. You should be ready for the next week on placement where the whole process will begin again.

If this feels an unnecessary and arduous task, remember that it is an essential part of your personal and professional development and will provide evidence of your progress as you continue through the course and throughout your career. It is vital to demonstrate how you are continuing to develop in order to maintain your professional registration, and highlight your competencies, so supervision is a skill which is equally as important to acquire as your practical ones, and like any skill the more you practice the easier it becomes.

Moving on after the supervision session

After the supervision session it is worth examining how you feel, breath deeply at this point. Supervision is designed to give you feedback on your performance so that you can pass the placement. If you receive some feedback that makes you feel uncomfortable, try to analyse it.

Box 8.5

1. List the areas that your educator told you were going well.

●

●

●

You can build on these, and if you cannot list anything here it is worth putting in the request for some positive feedback on your next supervision session and discussing this with your university liaison tutor.

2. List the areas that your educator might have suggested that you could improve on.

●

●

●

It is important that you relax and try not to leap immediately to your own defence, which we know is hard. Keep calm and try to analyse the areas again without being defensive, often this can be about perceptions or how each person has seen things. This can often become distorted on practice as there is the constant pressure of being assessed.

Example

A student comes away from a treatment session, which obviously was not perfect as it was only the student's first attempt. The student is asked to evaluate their performance by their educator, 'How do you think it went?'

The student, not wanting to highlight any deficits in performance and hoping that the educator did not notice any of small things that did not quite go to plan, says, 'Fine, I thought I did quite well, no problems really?'

As the educator, what would you think about the student's response?

To give you some idea about how an educator might respond to this, here are some thoughts that they might have in response to this situation:

'The student had little insight into their performance, which would worry me.'

'I would be concerned about their lack of ability to reflect on the session.'

'I would be anxious about the student's future development, how could they improve on their performance?'

How does that compare to your list?

Can you see how a small remark can cause unnecessary alarm bells to set off in your educator's mind? Over and over again, honesty is the best policy. Try to keep to the facts and the implications of them on your placement. Have another go at the supervision prep session as if you were this student and examine how you could move things on. How you could change the educator's perceptions of you and stop all those alarm bells from ringing. Remember, you have full access to the criteria that you are being marked against on your assessment form so use it to your advantage.

If things are still not going well

Try to think about it objectively. Think about it from the educator's point of view. Take responsibility for your actions and be clear about ways that you have suggested that you can improve during the following week. Read and work through Chapters 3 and 12 on reflection and failure. Bring some evidence of your reflections and talk these through during supervision. Come back to this chapter and identify what things you need to discuss as a result of your reflections in next week's supervision session.

Talk honestly to your educator and university liaison tutor, and try really hard not to compare yourself to other students. This is your professional journey, and like you and the objectives that you set with your educator during supervision, it is unique.

Chapter outcomes

Now that you have completed this chapter you should feel more confident to:

➡ identify your role in supervision
➡ develop an agenda for supervision
➡ discuss issues with your educator in supervision
➡ link strands of your ongoing personal and professional development to supervision and develop an action plan with objectives.

Further reading

Hawkins, P. and Shohet, R. (2000) *Supervision in the helping professions.* 2nd edn. Maidenhead: Open University Press.

Morrison, T. (2005) *Staff supervision in social care: making a real difference for staff and service users.* Brighton: Pavilion.

Stuart, C. (2003) *Assessment, supervision and support in clinical practice: a guide for nurses and other health professionals.* Edinburgh: Churchill Livingstone.

Van Ooijen, E. (2003) *Clinical supervision made easy.* Edinburgh: Churchill Livingstone.

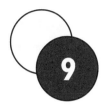

9 The personal and professional development process

- **Introduction**
- **Professional and course requirements**
- **Continuing professional development (CPD)**
- **An individual working and learning tool**
- **The content of a personal portfolio or progress file**
- **The personal and professional development process**
- **Employability**
- **The secret part!**
- **The process: capturing your learning and using it**
- **Finding out new things about yourself**
- **Self-awareness and PPDP**
- **Action plans**
- **Summary**

By the end of this chapter you will:

➡ be aware of the process of developing and integrating your placement learning
➡ have a format for recording your placement learning
➡ be able to identify transferable learning from placements
➡ be able to identify personal learning needs
➡ be able to write workable action plans to address your continuing learning needs.

Introduction

The personal and professional development process (PPDP) enables you to capture your own individual learning throughout the life of your course. You do this by:

➡ recording what you do
➡ reflecting on your learning
➡ identifying what else you need to do and how you are going to do these things.

It gives you the framework to capture your learning and develop the skills and knowledge that you individually need to develop. This is a part of all health and social care courses and the beginning of a process that will last throughout your career. In some courses the process is referred to as PPDP and portfolios are used, and in others it is addressed in what are known as 'Progress files'. We will discuss the formats later but what they all essentially cover is academic, placement and personal learning throughout the course.

For academic learning this is a relatively straightforward process: you have feedback from academic assignments and that should tell you some of what you need to do to improve your work. For instance, it may mean that you need to do more reading around a given subject or that you need to work on your critiquing skills or your referencing abilities. For placement learning it involves looking at the whole sum of your learning on placement, your theoretical knowledge and your ability to apply it, your practice skills and your personal learning and insight. You can see how this links in with the other chapters, but especially, Chapter 3 on reflective practice and Chapter 4 on setting learning objectives.

Professional and course requirements

Your course will require you to participate in this process of personal and professional development planning, but how you are asked to record this and whether it is assessed or not will depend on the individual programme of study. Some just require students to keep a progress file, to document this process; some require students to write assignments evaluating their personal and professional learning; while others require students to compile a portfolio of their learning over the course.

Continuing professional development (CPD)

The personal and professional development portfolio goes beyond the remit of your course, however. It will form part of your lifelong learning record and your evidence of continual professional development (CPD), which is a requirement of registration for all the health and social care professions. You can see how getting this right will be important to your whole career and not just your present course.

An individual working and learning tool

Although there will be many specific requirements of your course and your profession, the single most important factor about personal and professional development portfolios or progress files is that they are useful, workable documents for *YOU*. They are for you and about you so you need to feel happy with the process of what you are doing, and feel able to use the file to help you with your learning and development. You should control it, not it control you! This chapter will give you some ideas about what sorts of things can be included in it and the processes behind it, which will be relevant whatever your specific professional requirements. We want to make it a useful tool in your learning and your career development rather than another chore to do or hoop to jump through. Try to see it as an expression of you, who you are, what is important to you, where you want to go in your learning and your career, so that it is an expression of your individuality.

The content of a personal portfolio or progress file

Many people fall at the first hurdle because they cannot visualize what is wanted or required for a personal portfolio or progress file, so we will start with what it is. It is a paper or electronic file, or record of your learning of what you have done and engaged in during the course, including:

➡ what you have learnt from what you have done
➡ how you have reflected on or analysed your learning
➡ what you have identified as your learning needs and your strengths
➡ how you have planned to address those needs.

In order for it to be a useful and workable document, you will need to give it some structure so that you can know where to go to find things when needed. This may be either for yourself or if needed for tutorials and eventually, when you are applying for jobs and going for interviews.

There are many ways of structuring your file. The most important thing is that you find a structure that suits your style and the requirements of your course. However, here are some suggestions that can help you with this. Feel free to regard these as tips only and disregard anything that you do not think would work for you. There is not one perfect way of structuring your file, experiment and try different ways to challenge yourself until you find a way that suits your needs. Here are some simple tips:

❶ If you are working on paper, use a ring binder of some sort as it allows you to move things about as your priorities change and you move through your course.
❷ Designate part of your file for personal use only and the other part for public consumption, i.e., that you will show to your personal tutor, practice supervisor or mentor, or that you will hand in to be marked.
❸ Remember Chapter 3 on reflection. You can only get the most out of reflection if you are not censoring yourself.

❹ If you are writing what you know the tutor or supervisor wants to hear, you will not be totally honest and will not get the most learning out of the situation.

❺ If the file is to be a working document it will make sense to keep everything in there but have detachable sections which are just for your use only.

❻ **Remember that any information about service users must be anonymised so that confidentiality is maintained. No names or personal details about service users should be included in any part of the portfolio or file.**

Some universities have online packages that allow you to complete the PPDP completely electronically with access to web-based packages that guide you through the process, ask you to complete reflections and action plans and allow you to access your PPDP whenever you are at your computer. Other courses may have online tools and forms that you can complete and download and add to a paper PPDP. Your choice will be directed by the requirements of your course and the facilities available to you, but you may have a personal preference for a paper or an online file. Remember it is your file and you need to be able to feel comfortable using it and make it work for you.

Structuring your file

Whether you choose an online file or a paper file you will need to structure the sections in the file. If you are recording, reflecting and action planning on three or more years' work, you are going to need to order and organize the file so that it does not become too unwieldy. The file is a working document. As you go through the years of your course you will naturally deal with and move on from certain learning needs while others will be on-going. You need a system where you can archive anything that is no longer relevant to you and retain the parts that are still on-going or useful to your reflections. There are several ways you can do this, figure 9.1 provides a diagram of the process and an example of a structure.

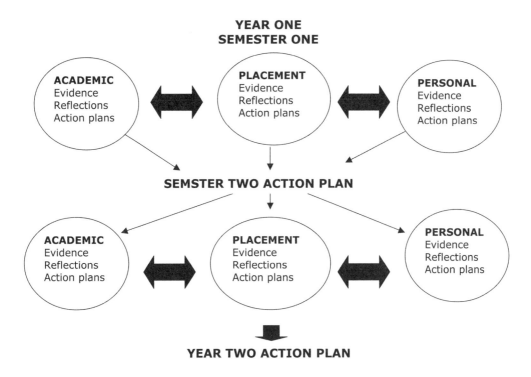

Figure 9.1

The personal and professional development process

It can often be bewildering to sort out what goes where in a PPDP file or portfolio. To begin with it pays to be structured and simple. That way you will know where to put things and where to find them. As you become more confident with the process you can move things around and link up recurring themes. It may help to have a series of prompts to ask yourself as you put information or evidence, such as feedback, into the file. This will help you make use of the feedback and take the next step to decide what you need to learn from it and do in the future. Figure 9.2 gives some basic ideas about how to organize the file and some prompts to help you reflect and action plan.

	SECTION 1 ACADEMIC	SECTION 2 PRACTICE	SECTION 3 PERSONAL
Record of achievement	• Formative feedback • Assignment feedback • Module evaluations	• Assessment form • Supervision records • Journal	Voluntary work Achievements Roles and responsibilities
Reflections on your learning	Reflections on feedback – what have I learnt? • What else do I need to know? • How does this fit in with my view of myself? • Why did it go well/not go well?	How do I feel about the placement and what I achieved? • What has been my biggest area of learning? • What went really well? • What was I not so happy about? • What else do I need to work on?	How have I developed as a person this semester? • What have I done that I am proud of and why? • What do I wish I had done and why? What stopped me from doing it? • What feedback am I getting from friends about myself?
Action Planning	What do I need to do? • Who can help me? • Where can I find the resources? • What am I going to do • When am I going to do it by? • How will I know when I have achieved it?	What do I need to do to take my learning forward? • What else do I need to find out about? • Where can I find the knowledge or gain the experience I need? • What am I going to do? • When am I going to do it? • How will I know when I have achieved it?	How can I develop more in the way I want to? • What can I do to expand my skills? • Who can help me with this? • Where can I go to do this? • What could I do? • When could I do it by? • How will I know when I have achieved it?

Figure 9.2

It may also be that by year two or three you want to organize your PPDP in a more subtle way, pulling together themes for learning which span all three domains: the personal, the academic and the placement arenas. For example, you could have three sections: 'self-direction', 'practical skills' and 'self-awareness', or other similar themes. These could easily transcend the boundaries of the academic, placement or personal divisions.

Employability

One of the most important aspects you will need to structure in to your PPDP in your final year is to make an explicit link between what you are learning in this year that prepares you for qualification and employment. You may want to make this explicit in the structure by adding a section after each subsection for you to list and reflect on how your learning is preparing you for employment; how the knowledge and skills you have gained are going to translate into the kinds of skills and knowledge that an employer will want.

The secret part!

This simple structure for capturing and keeping the PPDP, will make it a workable and usable document for you to progress and develop.

Do not forget the private section of this document, however. Give yourself one part or section where you can write or draw whatever you want, that you can remove before you show your file to anyone else. Use this section to be as creative as you want: mix and match your plans and thoughts; dream and doodle; use photographs. You may be surprised how many new ideas can come from letting your normal, careful guard down!

The process: capturing your learning and using it

The whole process is about making your learning *explicit*. Studying in health and social care courses demands a great deal of your time and attention. You can go from one module to the next without having time to catch your breath, and from one assignment to the next exam without having time to stop and think about what you are doing. When you get to the holidays, if you are lucky enough to have any, you are probably so exhausted you want to forget all about your course and just relax for a while. Studying like this it is very easy to miss vital learning points, to forget how you felt when you were doing something on placement and then studying it at university. You may make fleeting connections in your head at the time but if you do not capture them, in some form, that extra learning can be lost and you may not reap the benefits you could if you were able to give it more attention.

What the personal and professional development process does is engage you in capturing that learning so that you *can* benefit from it, and develop further. You can then articulate this learning to your advantage when you are applying for jobs and later, for promotion.

Example 1

Colin is a nursing student on a problem-based learning (pbl) course where much of the learning is self-directed and group work based. Small groups of students are given a scenario and they have to identify what they need to find out, go out and find out about it, and then share their knowledge and learning in order to achieve the task.

Colin has just finished one such module on the subject of rehabilitation nursing. He has just had feedback from the final case study assignment which he passed with a mark in the 50s. He is a little disappointed by the mark as he put a great deal of work into the module and the assignment. The main issue from the tutor's feedback is that he needs to focus more clearly on the assignment task and not to go off on a tangent. The tutor feels he has sacrificed depth for breadth.

Reflecting on this feedback Colin realizes that in the assignment he was trying to represent all the work that they had done in their pbl group during the module. He had been keen to demonstrate how widely they had researched the subject rather than concentrating on what had been asked of him in the assignment and applying this knowledge to this new scenario. He had been so caught up in the energy of the group that he had not stopped to analyse what was being asked of him in the assignment. He remembers the group sessions where they shared their thoughts and research and recognizes that, although they were enjoyable, they were also quite unfocused at times. There was a lot of excitement and energy around what they were doing but they never really structured the sessions and often ran over their time. Colin writes all this down in his reflections on the module and includes this in his PPDP file. As he is looking at all the work he has done this semester, he realizes there is a common theme across feedback from tutors and practice. He realizes that he may benefit from a more structured approach. He is able to incorporate this into his action plans for the next semester and decides to introduce more structure to the pbl group and to ask his next placement mentor about working in a more structured way.

This ability to help you integrate your learning is one of the most important aspects of the PPDP. Read the following example.

Example 2

Ester is a social work student returning from her second placement in a child and family centre, where she was involved in two complex child protection cases. She kept a reflective diary and has recorded some of her thoughts and learning from the situations. On return to university she attends a session on gender politics and during this a discussion on men and masculinity reminds her of an incident back in practice, where the father of one of the children became extremely aggressive towards his partner and her social work practice teacher (female). At the time Ester had 'written him off' as an abusive person and thought no more about him other than to register her fear and to make sure she was never alone with him. This session makes her think more about the man's behaviour and her own and her practice teacher's reaction to it. When she gets home that evening, Ester revisits her reflections on the incident and writes another piece about how the man's behaviour had the power to control them and how he may have learnt that behaviour from his past and his current social networks. She is not seeking to excuse his behaviour in any way, but sees that she needs to understand more about what was happening in that situation. She makes a note or action plan to find out about what services are available for men in this area. Can they access anger management or any types of therapeutic services if they were aware and wanted to change their behaviour? She concludes the piece of writing by identifying where she can go to find out more and makes a note to do a journal search for articles on men and masculinity and social work practice.

In this example, you can see how the act of capturing a piece of learning allows Ester to make links between her learning in placement and in study. She is able to make the links and take it further, that is to *develop* her learning.

Finding out new things about yourself

At the beginning of this book, in Chapter 2 about preparing yourself for the placement experience, it was suggested that it may help to do some self-assessments about how you rate your interpersonal skills, such as communication and assertiveness, for instance. These can provide a basis for the personal learning and development section of the PPDP. Throughout your course you will find out things about yourself that you may not have been aware of previously. The PPDP allows you to capture this new learning and use it in your academic and placement experience to enhance your overall learning and to enable you to articulate your development when it comes to job interviews. One of the most common job interview questions is, 'What have you learnt about yourself during your course?' The PPDP process can help you answer that question in a very real way with examples of how you have developed personally and professionally over the life of the course.

It is a useful exercise to start each semester/term and year with a 'check-up' analysis. You need to see where you feel you are at, what you want to achieve, what can help you reach those achievements and what can possibly stop you from achieving them. This is sometimes called a SWOT analysis. In a SWOT analysis you identify where your current strengths are (S); where your current weaknesses are (W); what opportunities you have (O), and what threats there are that might stop you achieving your aims (T). (The SWOT analysis was devloped by Albert Humphrey, who led a research project at Stanford University in the 1960s and 1970s.) There are several very straightforward ways of doing this, for example, dividing a piece of paper into four and labeling each section S, W, O and T– then listing relevant information below. See Figure 9.3 for an example of pre-placement SWOT analysis.

S (Strengths)	W (Weaknesses)
Anatomy knowledge – did well in last module. Area I like and feel very motivated. Good feedback from last placement. Confidence growing. Like the fast pace of this area. Near to home, not too much time travelling.	Brand new area – never done orthopaedics before. Will be only student there – not much peer support on site. I will be supervisor's first student.
O (Opportunities)	T (Threats)
Large teaching hospital so will have lots of different areas I can tap in to – particularly would like to see burns section. Have good lunch-time seminars and journal club for staff and students. Staff group have done a lot of research – could talk to them about this and see how I could incorporate it into my work.	Moving flats in the middle of the placement. Two pieces of academic work to be done as well as placement. It is going to be tiring as it is all new and there will be a lot of background reading and research to do in evenings. My girlfriend will be on placement as well – so we will both be needing support!

Figure 9.3

A SWOT analysis gives you a starting point from which you can identify what you may need to do to make the most of the opportunities facing you in a new semester or placement, or what you might need to do to make sure you get those opportunites.

Self-awareness and PPDP

Honesty and openness are the most crucial aspects of PPDP and if you want to learn about yourself you have to be open to challenge; from yourself as well as others. This is about acknowledging where you need to do more work, where you are not so good at something, but also, acknowledging where you *are* good at things and even where you excel at certain things. In this way you can harness your talents to develop the areas you want to improve.

If you are worried about being too honest because a tutor or mentor has to see your PPDP file and you think they may see you as 'lacking', do not worry. Any tutor or mentor will appreciate your honesty as long as you have looked at how and when you can deal with that issue. Whatever it is it will probably be picked up at some point in the course anyway, whether at university or on placement. The fact that you identify it yourself is a positive sign that you are taking responsibility for your learning and doing something about it. Demonstrating skills in self-awareness is a vital compentency in any health and social care professional. We all need to know what we do not know and where we need to develop more skills. Without this self-knowledge we could be dangerous practitioners.

Example

Lucy is a first year occupational therapy student who has completed four modules before going out on her practice placement. Before she arrives on placement, she is worried about what to put on her learning contract. Lucy knows she is a quiet person; she likes to listen more than talk. She looks back at the SWOT analysis she did at the start of the semester and the start of her course. In the analysis she identified her lack of confidence speaking in public as something that could stop her achieving what she wanted from the course.

She knows that she is going into a busy mental health team where they have twice weekly team meetings and is slightly scared about what they ask of her. She cannot imagine how she is going to feel if she is asked to report back on anyone at the meeting, for instance. She decides to do something about it and arrives at placement with the following learning objective already in her learning contract for the first half of the placement:

> Learning need: To develop confidence in verbal communication with team.
> Learning objective: To report to team on progress of at least one client.
> Resources needed: Support from placement educator in supervision.
> Practice reporting to placement educator.
> Timing: To report to team within first four weeks.
> Evidence: Feedback from team and educator.
>
> Lucy sets herself an achievable goal which can be developed further over the second half of the placement; she has incorporated the support of the placement educator and set up procedures to help herself along the way. She could have ignored this and just hoped that she would find the confidence she needed.
>
> When she returns from placement, she records what she has done in her PPDP file and reflects on how she felt about the challenge. She knows she still needs to do more to feel confident in talking to groups of people. She moves this forward again by action planning to speak to the next module leader and ask if she could do a ten-minute presentation on an aspect of her work on placement which is relevant to the module. The tutor concerned is very willing to incorporate this into one of the sessions and asks if others would like to do something similar. She congratulates Lucy on coming up with the idea. Lucy does the short presentation and asks for feedback from her tutor and fellow students. She now has more experience and more useful feedback to use to develop her skills still further. She could have chosen to ignore this aspect of herself altogether and suffer in silence but instead she has used the PPDP to challenge herself and develop her skills.

Action plans

Forming a realistic action plan is a crucial part of PPDP. Without it the process can just be a paper one. It is no use recording what you do, then identifying learning needs and development if you do not plan how to meet these needs in the future. There are several formats for structuring this process. Most of the formats available are similar to the learning contract style of: defining the learning need; setting the objective; and detailing what you need to achieve it and how you can achieve it realistically within a time frame. Look at your university's documentation on action plans and refer back to Chapter 4 on learning contracts to find a structure that suits your style of working and fits in with the requirements of your course.

The action planning process is not a separate add-on to the PPDP process – it is an on-going process that forms part of the basis for your next semester's or next year's planning.

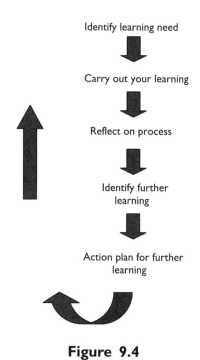

Figure 9.4

Action plans need to be living documents that are constantly reviewed. They not only look backwards to your reflection on what you have done and what that tells you, but they also look forward to what is going to be asked of you in the coming period of time. They also need to reflect your overall learning, from all domains, so that they reflect your development as a health and social care professional. Although you may want to make individual action plans for each section of your file, you will need to synthesize these with an overall plan for your future planned learning experiences. Read the following example:

Example

Robert is a final year physiotherapist student about to start his final semester before qualification. He has passed all his academic and clinical education modules so far. He has two more modules and his final research dissertation to complete.

From reflections on his last semester's work feedback, Robert has identified the following areas he needs to develop:

Academic:

➡ To incorporate more research evidence in assignment discussion.
➡ To introduce more critique and synthesis into his work.

Clinical education:

➡ Develop confidence in own abilities and convey this to clients.
➡ Be more pro-active in researching new and complex conditions.
➡ Develop more assertive and confident, professional manner.

Personal:

➡ Spend more time with others on his course.
➡ Get more involved in course activities.
➡ Give up part-time job to concentrate on study.

Robert incorporates these into an action plan, taking into account where he needs to be by the end of this semester.

Robert's final student action plan

Learning need: To be able to present myself at an interview as a competent, self-directed, responsible physiotherapist with an understanding and commitment to life-long learning. To make the transition from student to newly qualified practitioner.

Robert's learning objectives/action plan for this semester

➡ Synthesize my learning so far and develop a CV and reorganize PPDP file to present at interview.
➡ Practise interview techniques with peers and tutors. Research possible interview questions, practise with friends and peers, gain feedback from peers and tutor on my performance.
➡ Develop my skills in finding and using research for all areas of my work. Book sessions in library with learning support unit using draft outline of module assignment. Identify relevant research evidence; work through research critiquing tools to identify most useful for my purpose.
➡ Read and download relevant government policy and directives for clinical practice in my area.
➡ Consult student support services for possible assertiveness training courses.
➡ Employ time management techniques to allocate time to each module and assignment.
➡ Organize physio social events this semester!

At the end of this semester and the course, Robert would then adapt his action plan to reflect the transition to working in practice by looking at what the requirements of his specific new job will be.

Summary

The PPDP process allows you to capture and analyse all aspects of your learning throughout your course and on to your first job. It gives structure to a process that may otherwise be subconscious and therefore inaccessible. It allows you to benefit from your learning and be able to articulate your learning to yourself, your tutors and placement supervisors and, finally, your would-be employers.

The process involves recording your learning, reflecting on it and then identifying and planning for further learning needs. It can be done on paper or online, but it is ultimately only of use to you if you can *use* it so you need to find a format that meets your needs and those of your course and professional body. The key to a useful and productive PPDP file is for you to be honest with yourself about your learning.

Chapter outcomes

Having read this chapter you should now be able to:

➡ understand the process of recording, reflecting and action planning
➡ have an idea of how to format your PPDP file
➡ understand how to use the process to integrate your learning
➡ understand how to use the process to develop your employability.

Further reading

Hull, C. and Shuttleworth, A. (2005) *Profiles and portfolios: a guide for health and social care* 2nd edn. Palgrave and Macmillan.

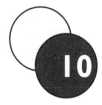

10 Interprofessional perspectives on placements

- **The service user**
- **Mrs Richardson's story**
- **Knowing our roles and working together**

By the end of this chapter you will be able to:

➡ identify interrelationship between professional roles in the placement area
➡ consider the importance of interprofessional communication from the points of view of the service users and carers
➡ highlight potential common ground between the professionals
➡ highlight barriers to potential interprofessional working
➡ identify good interprofessional working practice.

If we want to provide the best service we can to service users, no matter what our own professional role, we must all put the service user at the centre of everything we do. You will be a student on placement for a given length of time; the service user is also there for a given length of time. The professionals working in the service may have been there for a few years, or several years, but they will certainly be the best people there. This can be a very positive thing. The professionals are the experts who will have a vast amount of specialist knowledge of the area and local knowledge about related services; they will know how it all works and how it all fits together. It can also, however, have a down side if the professionals working there forget what their services look like to people from the outside and if they forget to explain how it all works.

The service user

You know as a student what it feels like to start a new placement when you know very little about where you are going and what is going to be asked of you; it can be very stressful. Now imagine what it must feel like for the service user, who does not know much about the service and may also know very little about their 'condition' or needs or even what is happening to them. They do not know how the services all fit together, who does what, what is expected of them and what they can expect from the service.

You can see immediately how important it is to make sure that the service user is aware of what is happening and what is likely to happen to them. Communication has to start between students and professionals as the ones who know the service. Once you have a good communication system working, where everyone has a common understanding and purpose, it is much easier to convey this to service users. In doing this you can help put them at the centre of their treatment or services, which is exactly where they should be.

You will rarely be working in a uni-professional environment. Depending on where you are placed you could be working with a number of key professions who will be part of the service user's treatment or service.

Box 10.1 What do you know of other professionals' roles?

| How would you describe the role of the following? |
| Who do you think they would work with? |
| Where do you think they work mostly? |
| A nurse |
| A physiotherapist |
| A social worker |
| An occupational therapist |
| A radiographer |
| Do any of these roles overlap? |
| What common skills do they all need? |

Whatever your knowledge of other professions, you should be able to recognize that there is a great deal of common ground among these professionals: who they work with, where they work and even in what they do. Is it not interesting, then, that it is often our differences that we concentrate on so defensively! Within a hospital setting you would probably see all the above professionals. For example, if an older person was admitted to hospital following a fall and they were found to be unable to cope at home any more, it would be highly likely that *all* of the above professionals would come into contact with this person. How do you think they can best work together to ensure that the client they have in common receives the best treatment?

Read the following fictional diary extract and think about how our interprofessional communication systems impact on the quality of the experience of the service user.

A morning in the life of Mrs Richardson

Patient on Ward C (rehabilitation), Northern Counties General Hospital.

Mrs R is on a fast rehab ward following a treatment for a fractured neck of femur and a Colles fracture. She is also recovering from a chest infection. Mrs R is 78-years old and was previously enjoying reasonably good health.

Monday 7am

I am woken by the staff coming on duty. They always have a meeting about this time. I think they let the day staff know how everybody's been in the night – at least that's what it sounds like. I heard them talking about me one morning, soon after I was transferred here. They were a bit worried that I might be confused. I think they said I had been rambling a bit in the night. I meant to tell them that I have always talked in my sleep. My husband used to complain about it all the time we were married. Didn't tell them in the end as I thought they would be annoyed if they knew I could hear what they said.

7.30 Dorothy, the domestic lady brings me my breakfast, just a slice of toast and another cup of tea, I don't like to eat or drink too much because getting to the loo is still difficult. They think I'm just a very light eater. Little do they know what I can put away at home!

8.30 The OT – this stands for occupational therapist – and her student arrive. Sue, the OT, had come up to see me on Friday to tell me she would be coming, I remembered when I saw her. She introduced her student. She looks so young, she can't be more than 16 surely and Sue asked if I would mind if the student helped as well as she has to learn. I said I didn't mind, but I do of course. It's bad enough that I have to try to get dressed in front of one stranger never mind two, still what could I say? I want to be helpful and I want to get out of here. She said it wasn't a test and she wanted to help me be able to do everything for myself again. This is the first time I have tried to get dressed in nearly a week and a half now. I feel so stupid. Sue had to rummage through my things to find my clothes. I don't know why she didn't just let me do it myself and then I could tell her what the problems were. She was very nice about it and she offered to help me when I got stuck with things like my tights. She even offered to give me some equipment to help but really I don't care that much. I could just wear slippers for a while until I get better. I can keep the heating on at home and I won't need tights!

I just want to get out of here. I managed to stand alright and she showed me how to get a bra on by having it done up and stepping into it. Hilarious really, if I didn't feel so stupid. I almost started crying at one point; there I was trying desperately to hook a pair of knickers round my feet, while these two young women stood on looking at me. Sue was very jolly about it though, so that made me get on with it.

Then she asked me a lot of questions about my house and what I do with myself at home. She asked me if I had thought of having my bed downstairs as it would be much safer. I laughed and she looked at me a little strange, but why would I want a bed downstairs when I have a fantastic bedroom with a lovely new double bed and a view over the hills out of the window. I love sitting up in bed in the morning looking out over the sky and the hills. She went through a lot of questions. I'm sure I told them all this when I first came in but maybe they didn't get through to the other departments. Anyway she seems to think I will be fine in a few days and so I should be able to be home by the end of the week, if not before.

9.30 A porter came and told me to get ready to go down to physio. I didn't even know I was going this morning. I hadn't been down on Friday or on Saturday or Sunday, but I don't think they work at weekends. Luckily, I was dressed this time. Last time I had to go down in my nightie and dressing gown. I felt very embarrassed being wheeled along those corridors with all those people in their outdoor coats walking past.

Angela was waiting for me in physio. She looked at my feet and started to tut tut. She said I shouldn't be wearing my slippers and that I wasn't steady enough. She seemed a bit annoyed but I didn't know that I was coming to physio this morning. If I had known I would have asked Sue to get my trainers out. I had them brought in specially, but never mind. She said we would have to work in a carpeted room so she took me off to a little room with a bed in it. She asked me to get out of the wheel chair and use a frame. My wrist really hurt but I had to use it otherwise I would have toppled over. It was really hard to grip the frame because it seemed so high but I managed. It was like the one they had given me on the ward but it didn't have wheels. I did all she asked me, walking around, turning with it, but when I let slip that the one on the ward was much smaller and had wheels she seemed very annoyed and asked who had given it to me? I couldn't remember and she said she would find out. She let me sit down after a while and she filled in some paperwork. She started to ask me the same sorts of questions as Sue the OT had done earlier, all about my house and what sorts of things I did during the day. When I told her that Sue had just asked me these very same things she seemed to be surprised. I don't know why but I don't think she liked me saying that. Anyway she said she thought I was doing really well too and that it wouldn't be long before I was home. I wasn't in physio very long.

11am Made it back to the ward, after a bit of a wait for a porter. I was tired after all this so had a bit of a nap in my chair but I was woken abruptly by one of the nurses, I think it was Helen. She said that the consultant was coming round and I had better be awake! I asked her if it meant that I could go home and she just raised her eyebrows and looked blank. I don't think she knew really. The consultant started making his way around the ward. He had three or four other younger looking doctors with him and two of the nurses were with them as well. They didn't spend much time with anyone really and they were talking quite quietly so I couldn't get a feel for what it was all about. When they got to me they gathered around the bed and he looked at my wrist and asked me to move my fingers and grip his hand. He then asked me to get up out of the chair, well I'd only just woken up from my nap and after all the commotion this morning I was a bit stiff so it took me a bit longer than it had done earlier. He looked at Helen, who I think is the nurse in charge and said something about a nursing home – I know he did – I distinctly heard him – even though he wasn't talking to me. Well I went red in the face I could feel it, I shouted at him, 'I'm not going into a nursing home, I won't, I've got my own house and I can cope. You can't put me in a nursing home!' I was really, really upset. It's the one thing I dread and I just couldn't bear it. Well he just looked at me as if I was mad and walked away. I was furious. Helen stayed behind and told me not to worry. She said he didn't mean going to live in one, just go for a bit of 'intermediate care' or something like that she said. She couldn't stop with me, she had to follow him to finish his round, so I was left there absolutely scared stiff. They had all said I was doing well, that I would probably be home soon. Now what was this? I just couldn't help crying. I cried and cried at the very thought of it. Helen sent a student nurse over to talk to me. I saw her pointing at me and this little lass came up and sat on my bed with me. She was lovely really; she held my hand, not in a patronizing way, but in a lovely warm supportive way. She told me about this intermediate care. It seems like they've moved some of the hospital staff out there. It's just like being in hospital but it's not a hospital it's a residential home but people from the hospital are in a separate part of it. They have nurses and OTs and physios she said. She'd been out to see it last week and she thought it was nice, better food she said. I was a bit reassured by her but why couldn't they have told me earlier? She said that loads of people from here go to stay there and that rehab was done there. No-one told me that. She sat with me for at least 15 minutes and I felt much better after that but they brought the lunch round and I just couldn't eat it.

Think about some of the following questions

 At what point in this story did communication start to go wrong?

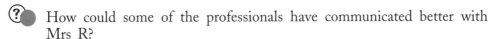

- How could some of the professionals have communicated better with Mrs R?
- What information could have been talked through with Mrs R?
- How were decisions made on this unit?
- What is the effect of bad communication on the service user?
- What examples of good communication were there in this story?
- What identifies them to you as good communication examples?

Mrs Richardson's story

From the above account we can feel immediately how alien an environment a hospital ward can be to someone who is not used to being there. Mrs Richardson does not know the rules and routines, the roles and procedures like the staff do. She tries to guess what is happening and make sense of it as best she can. She has her own agenda and that is to get better and get home as soon as she possibly can and in order to do this she feels she has to be a 'good' patient and comply with everything that is asked of her.

The ward system is organized around an efficiency-based process that allows all the staff to function in their roles. The ward is not organized around the needs of individual patients and so they can find it very difficult to understand how and why things are done as they are. One of our common roles as health and social care professionals is to communicate well with the people using the service. There are many ways in which we can do this. Written information on ward procedures can be given to people so they know what to expect. Each professional should take time to explain their role and the likely input they will have to the care of the patient. In this story the occupational therapist explained what she would be doing and requested permission to bring the student occupational therapist with her.

As well as having a duty to explain your role and input, if you think about the overall experience of Mrs Richardson, in order to ensure quality care is given, the individual professions have a duty to communicate with each other. In this story if the professionals involved, such as the occupational therapist, the physiotherapist and the nursing staff, had spoken more to each other, Mrs Richardson would have known that she was going to physiotherapy and needed her shoes and would be using the appropriate walking frame on the ward. Later on in the story we see how if the medical staff had communicated better and before they went to see Mrs Richardson, someone could have talked to her about intermediate care instead of which she was very upset and worried about the possibility of being sent to a nursing home.

How we, as professionals, communicate with each other is also important from another aspect. If we do not have good working practices and communication systems, it can mean that service users are asked unnecessary and sometimes inappropriate questions about information that has already been given. We saw this in the story when the physiotherapist and the occupational therapist were duplicating questions. Mrs Richardson has no notion of how these professions work together or how they keep their notes and she is rightly not interested. All she knows is that she is in hospital and she has already told someone this so why would someone else be asking her the very same question?

Systems to share information between professionals involved in someone's care are very important. These are improving all the time and multi-disciplinary notes are commonplace, however it is worth noticing as a student how often you read or look at other professionals' notes. Your role as a temporary 'visitor' to the setting can be utilized again to explore interprofessional communication. When you are discussing the service with your supervisor or mentor it is a good topic to debate and give constructive feedback: When have you seen it working well? Are there ways you think it could be improved?

As a student on placement one of the most useful things you can do to supplement your own professional learning is to arrange to spend time with other professionals. You can learn more in a few hours shadowing a colleague in their job than you can reading up for hours on professional roles. You will see how they work and what they do first-hand and you can then use this information to better your own practice. Your referrals on to other services will be more appropriate; you can re-enforce the different aspects of treatment a person is receiving from the other professionals involved and generally improve your patient or client's well-being by being able to explain their care. They will respect and trust you more for that and you will subsequently be able to work better with your client because of this.

In many health and social care placement sites there will often be a range of students on placement at the same time. If they do not already have one, why not suggest they run interprofessional student support groups or have interprofessional seminars for students on site?

Knowing our roles and working together

Giving the service user the best service you can does not solely rely on your own professional skills. You can be the best nurse, physiotherapist, social worker in the area and still the service user will not get the best service or treatment unless you understand what else they are going through, what other treatment or services they are accessing, who is involved in this and how that impacts on what you are doing.

If the professionals involved are not working together you can unwittingly be at odds with each other. One person may be advising one thing and another something completely different. This is why you spend the time you do at those meetings where people's cases are discussed between the team and where people agree on the direction that they are working towards as a team with a service user. As the student attending such meetings, it is very interesting to observe the power balances in such interprofessional teams. Try writing a reflective account of one of these multi-disciplinary meetings, looking at who wields the power and why and starting to analyse the communication issues among the team. How does the team deal with conflicting opinion? Who runs the meetings and sets the agendas?

What happens between meetings? What communication systems are in place on a day-to-day basis?

Box 10.2

Think of a service user you have worked with on placement.

(?) How many other professional were involved in the case – from start to finish and who were they?

(?) How did you communicate what you were doing with these other professionals?

(?) How do you think the service user benefited from this communication or not?

None of us work alone in these types of services. Even in specialist areas you will always need to be aware of related services that the service user can access and benefit from. At times we may need to put aside our own professional perspective and take a broader view of the overall care that the service user is receiving. If our input is going to be the best that we can give, it must fit in with the overall approach and care, so that the service user's experience is foremost in our practice.

Chapter outcomes

Having read this chapter you will now:

➡ have thought through some of the other professional perspectives
➡ have considered the service through the eyes of the service user
➡ have thought through the importance of good interprofessional communication.

Further reading

Barrett, G. (2005) *Interprofessional working in health and social care: professional perspectives.* Palgrave Macmillan.

Day, J. (2006) *Interprofessional working: an essential guide for health and social care professionals.* Cheltenham: Nelson Thornes.

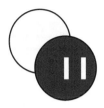

Evidence-based practice

- **Introduction**
- **Why the need for evidence-based practice?**
- **Theory and practice**
- **Specialist information and using the Internet**
- **Policy and practice – local and government websites**
- **Final year placements**
- **Support for your placement learning**
- **Summary**

By the end of this chapter you will be able to:

➡ understand the role of research and evidence-based practice in your practice learning
➡ identify sources of evidence to support your placement learning
➡ identify areas to investigate to widen your learning
➡ use the Internet for professional information and support
➡ use the Internet to build understanding of the context of placement learning and service user perspectives.

Introduction

You are ultimately on your placement to learn by doing. But doing is not just a matter of copying your supervisor or mentor. You will instead be combining learning from example, both with theoretical knowledge and reflection on the practical experience you accrue. Your theoretical knowledge is not left at university. You now need to make the theory fit the reality of the placement situation!

When out on your practice placement, your learning materials are very different from those which you have been used to at university. Do not forget, however, those university resources are still going to be very useful to you in your placement learning. You may be lucky enough to have online access to learning centre materials or you may be placed somewhere where online access is limited. If you are living away in accommodation you may not have access to your university learning centre at all or indeed Internet access in your accommodation or office. You need to be resourceful as a student and locate and utilize all the learning materials around you, even if this may mean finding the local library in your study time. In this chapter we will outline some ways in which you can locate and utilize useful information and the evidence base for the practice in which you are now participating.

Why the need for evidence-based practice?

Since the modernization programme for the NHS and social care began in the late 1990s, there has been an emphasis on accountability and clinical governance. Service users should be able to expect the same quality of care wherever they are treated and by whomever they are treated. This has led to the development of audit and best practice guidelines for most areas of services. As a practitioner you need to be able to demonstrate that your interventions are both effective and the best that can be expected by the service user. Experiential knowledge is no longer enough of a justification for doing something. Knowing something works is important but it is not enough. You need to know why and how something works and in what circumstances it does not. You need to know the context of your interventions, the protocols and programmes that your service is signed up to, and the government directives that guide them. As a student on placement the evidence base for the service is not your responsibility, that is for the service managers and providers to establish. You can, however, play a very important role in using evidence to develop and promote best practice and enhance your own learning.

Theory and practice

At university you will have become accustomed to using theory and research articles to underpin your discussions in written assignments. In practice settings many health and social care professionals find it difficult to find the time to discover and explore the evidence and research for some of the practice in which they are involved. Some practitioners have a remit specifically to do this, while others try to integrate it into an already very busy working week.

One of your roles, particularly in your final year as a student, can be to address the issues of research in practice. You are unlikely to have a full workload compared to your educator/mentor and you may well have computer and Internet access to your university websites and intranet. How could you play a part in embedding evidence-based practice within your service area while enhancing your learning at the same time?

Example

Padma is a final year nursing student starting a placement on a children's ward in an acute hospital. As part of her placement she needs to do a project on a new initiative. Padma has a special interest in health promotion and wants to look into this. She uses the Internet to get started by searching the Department of Health's website for policy on the subject. When she has looked at the national service framework for children and seen some of the policies that may be relevant, she also finds links to other projects across the country with a health promotion slant. She then goes on to her university intranet and does a literature search using Medline, Assia and Cinhal to establish what research has been done around this area of work.

This gives Padma a base line of ideas from which to start. She can then analyse this information to put together some suggestions for what might be most useful in her specific location. When she comes to her supervision session with her nursing mentor, she is able to give some solid justification for her ideas and the mentor is extremely interested. Padma offers to show her the articles and information about other such projects that she has found.

By approaching it in this way, Padma's project can lead to real and sustainable changes in practice, rather than just being something for university that she has to do to pass the placement.

On your placements your critique of practice and theory should be an integral part of the content of your supervision sessions and will develop in depth as you go through the three years of your course.

Evidence is not just research based, however. Service evaluations and audits can provide important information and statistics to guide practice and service provision and you may be involved in this on placement in some way too.

Your approach to using the theory in your practice area is important. You need to be realistic and pragmatic about how much of it you can reasonably hope to use in your given setting. Your placement supervisor will not be impressed if you are continually coming up with wonderful ideas of what could be done if only the service had more money or more staff. You need to be aware of the local factors that would make change and new practice feasible, or not. Here are two tips to get you started:

➡ Whenever you go out on a new placement, check the Department of Health and Social Care Institute for Excellence websites (http://www.dh.gov.uk and http://www.scie.org.uk/) for information about the types of services you are going in to. What are the most recent government policies in the area you will be in?
➡ Do a literature search on the relevant databases to discover what seem to be the key issues for research in the area you are going to. Even if you only read the abstracts before you go, you will gain an insight into some of the most current issues which may affect your service.

Specialist information and using the Internet

Web-based resources are an additional source of information and ideas to enhance your overall learning experience on placement and to integrate your theoretical learning with your placement learning. There is a wealth of viewpoints, experiences, ideas and knowledge which, used wisely, can assist you in understanding the complexities of a given situation or condition, and the government and local policies behind the services you work in. It can take you from the broad over-riding philosophy to the minute detail. The downside is that you need to feel confident navigating your way through the myriad sites that any searches can bring. You need to focus and use good time management skills in using the Internet to avoid becoming sidetracked.

Used well, you can tap in to the Internet not just for research evidence, as discussed above, but also for the following:

➡ *Policy and practice* – government websites for up-to-date information on policy and the background
➡ *Support for your placement learning* – using learning support networks and professional body websites
➡ *Other perspectives* – service user sites for information and narratives.

The guiding rule of using the Internet in your learning, both in the practice and academic settings, is to verify the status of the information you find. You must be able to distinguish between different types of information; for example, from anecdote, service user experience, government document, research-based papers and practice-based expert opinion. It is very important that you can do this and that you can use the right type of information in the right way. For instance, a paper written by someone with the title 'Professor', published on a random website is not necessarily going to be a reliable document. You will need to establish where the paper comes from, where the 'Professor' is working and if the paper has been peer reviewed in order for you to establish that it is from a bona fide professor and that the paper has been reviewed and therefore judged to be of an acceptable standard.

Similarly, you may come across a website from a self-help group that includes a number of stories about people's experiences in accessing mental health services.

While these can be illuminating in terms of their experience (see below) you cannot generalize from this that their experience is applicable to everyone in that situation. It may be, however, that this information will help you to ask questions of your own service and practice. Always verify your sources.

Policy and practice – local and government websites

In any placement setting, when you are working with any service user, what you do and how you do it will be determined by a combination of your professional remit and local policy about how the services are organized, prioritized and delivered. If you just confine your learning to what is done in your practice setting, without enquiring into the reasons behind the way the service is organized, you will only be learning on one level. If you understand the reasons behind the service organization and priorities you can make informed decisions about how you operate within that service, and you can also go the extra mile and be proactive in service development.

Example

Jane is an occupational therapy student on a placement in a community mental health setting. The service has been through many changes recently and the team are coping with a new way of working and a new system of allocating referrals within the team. Jane is trying to understand the system and talks to her placement educator about why they, as occupational therapists, get certain referrals and not others and why they prioritize certain ones above others. She thinks she understands this but is still confused sometimes at referral meetings. There are instances in referral meetings when nurses take on new assessments that Jane thinks should be taken by them as occupational therapists and she struggles to understand the reasoning for this.

In a quiet half-hour Jane looks on the Department of Health website to find out about new approaches to mental health services and new ways of working within those services. From reading the white papers and green papers, which are all helpfully in easily downloadable summaries, she is able to see the bigger picture and see where her team and her role fits in to this bigger picture. Now, instead of the issue seeming to be about individuals within her team and questions about 'Who does what?' she understands that the real issue is actually about changing professional roles and responsibilities, and that the needs of the service users are paramount. From her own research, she is able to take her new understanding of the situation further, reflecting on the implications of the changes on the new services and her role as an occupational therapist within that. She realises that social inclusion is a cross-professional role and one that all mental health practitioners must make central to their work. This means that traditional criteria for different professionals being allocated certain referrals has shifted fundamentally.

She brings this up at supervision and her placement educator is impressed with her grasp of what is behind the changes in the team. They are able to hold a challenging and informative discussion about the developing role of the professions and Jane is able to include this in her PPDP file as evidence of professional reflection backed up by government documents.

These days it is not enough to know your own clinical area and the practical and theoretical knowledge that underpins your approach. You will also need to have a grasp of the organization, foundations and philosophy of the service within which you will practice. As a physiotherapy student, for instance, going out on a placement in a unit for people with neurological conditions, it is not enough to read up on the conditions and the physiotherapy input and techniques. To work effectively within that department you will need to familiarize yourself with, for example, the national service framework for long-term (neurological) conditions. From this you can find out about initiatives in this area to develop good practice and information about how services have been developed across the country. You can now think about how this is translated in to practice in the area of your placement and perhaps how this could be developed further.

The Department of Health and the Social Care Institute for Excellence websites will be invaluable sources of information for you. They both also have many documents and publications, links to other sites and are generally mines of information for anyone working in health and social care. Take some time to familiarize yourself with them throughout your course but they become more and more important as you progress and make the transition from student to becoming a health and social care professional.

Final year placements

Final year placements demand a greater understanding of theory and research and it is worth pointing out that you would not perhaps be expected to incorporate as much theory and research into your early placements, where you are very much picking up and learning about new skills and concentrating on the practical. However, even at this early stage, it would be beneficial to make a habit of reading around your area. While buying textbooks will help you with the theory, knowing what else happens in practice in other parts of the country and the world will also enhance your overall practice learning. Remember that on placement you are not just learning how to do something, you are learning about the processes of doing certain things and how to apply those skills in a range of contexts.

Support for your placement learning

There are different places you can look for support online when on placement. Here we run through a few ideas.

Online discussion forums

Away on placement you may feel isolated from your usual support networks that you have at university. You may even have to live away from your usual base to go out on placement. There are many ways in which the Internet can help you stay in touch with your course tutors and your fellow students. Many of you will have web-based learning tools already in place with discussion boards for your use. On placement these can be doubly useful to you in keeping you in touch but also as another source of information. If you are unsure about some procedures or processes about the placement, for instance, you could use the discussion board as a first point of call. It may be useful to you if you feel there is something you want to know but dare not ask your placement educator/mentor. The benefits to using a group discussion board, as opposed to individually emailing your tutors, is that all your fellow students can benefit from the questions and answers. There are always issues about placement learning that people need to clarify and using the discussion board can benefit many students in one go. For this reason it is useful to keep checking the discussion boards because often other people's questions can pre-empt your own.

You can take this concept further and set up more co-operative learning groups.

➡ you can do this across student cohorts, so that you share with your student group some of the things you are learning
➡ you can do it across professions to develop your interprofessional learning
➡ you can do it across student years so that, for instance, other students from your profession who have been to that placement can help you with issues that may occur in that practice area
➡ you can build up a resource for students going to your placement in the future.

Online discussion boards have great potential for sharing learning, benefiting from other people's experience and developing your interprofessional knowledge and skills.

Professional body websites

These are a source of very useful information, both professional and clinical or practice based. They can alert you to current relevant issues as well as involve you in professional development discussions. These sites are an important place for you to contribute to your profession whether by joining special interest group discussions or giving feedback about your practice experience to your professional body. Many of your own professional codes of conduct and ethics will be on these websites and will be useful reference points at times in placement when complex decisions have to be made.

Web etiquette and discussion boards

With this sort of informal knowledge sharing online there does need to be some agreed web etiquette. It is notoriously easy to offend others by email! Written communication is generally typed off at speed, and of course is sent without the facial expressions or voice tones that can soften or ease what we are saying were we to say it verbally. Written words on a computer screen can be interpreted in very different ways from which they were meant, often depending on the state of mind of the reader. The language you use should be professional at all times and show respect for other people's views.

While it is useful to have a forum to air your views, you must always distinguish when you are expressing a point of view or an opinion only. Placements can be stressful experiences if you have had some difficulties either with people or processes. Web-based discussion forums are not the place to air grievances about supervisors or places. These should be dealt with on an individual basis with your tutors.

Confidentiality is also an issue to be clear about while discussing placement issues on these discussion boards. Just leaving out a client's or a supervisor's name is not enough and does not ensure confidentiality. Readers may well be able to deduce whom you are talking about just from knowing where you were on placement. A reader must not be able to trace back anyone you discuss.

Other wider discussion forums can also be a source of support and information. These range from profession-based discussion forums (see your profession's website) from international forums (see Yahoo groups) to interprofessional clinical or practice area discussions. These types of forum can give you ideas and widen the context of your thinking about your profession.

Online mentoring

This is another avenue you and your university may want to pursue to support you in placement learning or throughout your course. It can be extremely helpful to have someone who is not ever going to assess you, who is there only to support you, who you can email whenever you want to discuss something without the fear of being judged for how little or much you know. It could be final year students mentoring first year ones or it could be recent graduates or senior professionals supporting students through their course. Having this support online means that you can have another avenue of advice and guidance and another resource of wisdom to approach when you need it.

Other people's perspectives

The Internet connects you with a myriad of different perspectives on a subject. If you use it wisely you can harness these other perspectives to add to your understanding of the complexity of human experience that you come across on placement. One of the ways in which this can increase your placement learning is if you can learn from other people's experience of using the services in which you are on placement. The Internet is full of people's stories and these can range from individual websites and blogs to service user organization sites to major charities and voluntary service sites. Reading or listening to someone's experience of going through an illness or difficult time in their life can enhance our understanding of a situation and build on our empathy. We learn about what it was like to experience it from their point of view rather than our own. On the Internet these stories can often be accompanied by video and photographs that can make this even more real than reading texts or novels (see Chapter 2 on preparing yourself for placement). There are many educational and informational websites around where people's experiences of specific health conditions have been collected and are presented as a resource for learning for service users and professionals. Often these accounts can tell us about all the 'side issues' of having a certain illness that we as health care professionals may not take time to consider, for instance, many of the accounts recall the waiting times and places, the days between a test and a diagnosis, what it feels like to be undergoing tests for a life-threatening disease. These parts of the illness experience can be very influential in how a service user approaches treatment. If we as health and social care professionals are aware of them it can enhance our interactions with people as we understand more of what they are going through.

Service user websites, charities and voluntary services sites

These types of sites present organized information for other people and professionals and as such they can be useful to recommend to service users as well as for using yourself. Many large organizations, for instance, Alzheimer's Disease Society, NSPCC and Age Concern, have very informative, well signposted sites that are a mine of information on all aspects of their 'issue'. They can put you in touch with other professionals, local projects and funding, as well as being a reliable source of facts and statistics. As campaigning organizations they can be inspiring for you and empowering for service users so they can be of direct use in your practice.

There are several other sources that can provide you with useful insights to your practice area and the people you will come in contact with on placement. Radio programmes, for instance, that capture people's experience of illness and life problems can similarly be helpful in adding to your understanding and as an information source for you and service users. Radio programmes can often be accessed on the Internet and downloaded on podcasts to listen to again at your convenience.

Figure 11.1 Using the internet to support placement learning

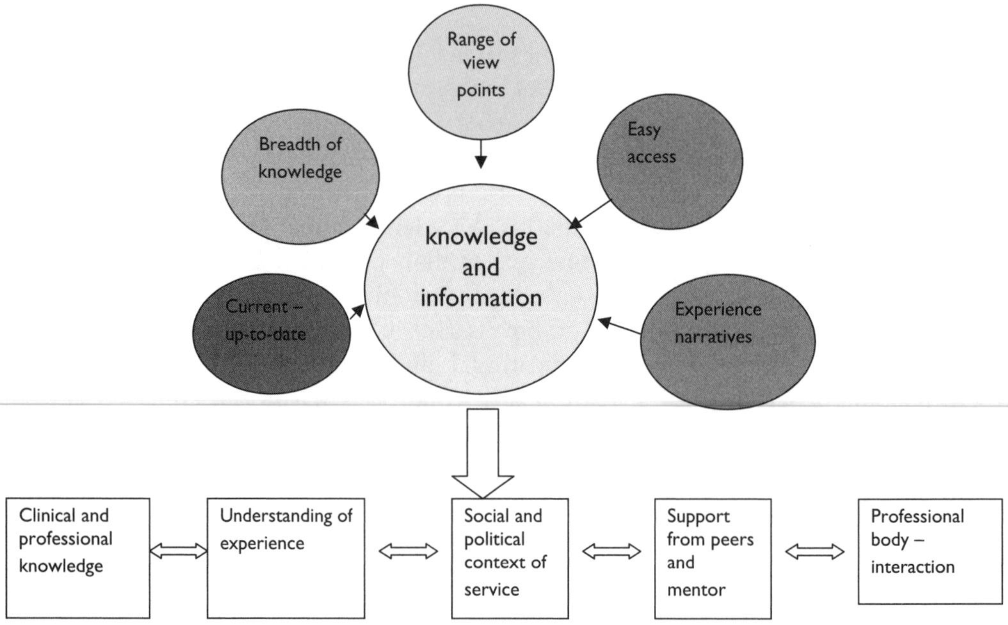

Summary

We have looked at how you can start to incorporate evidence-based information into your placement learning and how to develop your learning through accessing online resources. In this way you can better understand the complexities of the service you are working in and the experiences of the people you are working with.

The guiding principles for using the Internet are:

➡ focus – using your time wisely to concentrate on your subject and not getting sidetracked
➡ establishing the reliability and status of your sources and hence applying the information appropriately
➡ developing an interactive support network where your contributions can aid a co-operative learning environment.

Further reading

Corby, B. (2006) *Applying research in social work practice*. Maidenhead: Open University Press.

Craig, J. and Smythe, (2002) *The evidence based practice manual for nurses*. Edingburgh: Churchill Livingstone, L.

Taylor, M.C. (1999) *Evidence based practice for occupational therapists*. Oxford: Blackwell Science.

12 Failure

- **Thoughts and feelings**
- **Failing at the halfway point – what now?**
- **What if I don't get on with my placement educator?**
- **Failing the resit**

By the end of this chapter you will be able to:

→ explore failure, take it apart and put it back together again
→ identify your thoughts and feelings around failure and its implications for your future practice
→ prepare for your supervision sessions and halfway/final report
→ move on after failing a placement.

If we were to distil all the anxieties about placement we would probably be left with failure as the biggest single anxiety. If you are reading this chapter you may be either failing a placement or just be one of the many students who worries about failing a placement. Before we go any further, let us get the whole thing into some kind of perspective. If you were to fail your driving test (or any other test), as many of us do, you would probably be fairly philosophical about it. You would identify where you had gone wrong, acknowledge that you had tried hard to remember and do everything right but on this occasion had not quite managed it. Before long you would be ringing up for another test date. Keeping this perspective about placements is essential if you are going to:

→ listen to the feedback from your educator
→ reflect objectively on the feedback you receive
→ act on the feedback.

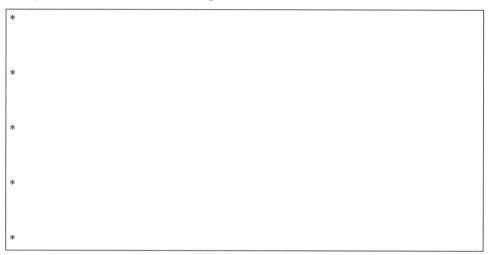

BOX 12.1

Why do you think that is difficult to maintain objectivity about failing a placement?

Try to write at least four things.

*

*

*

*

*

This is a good start. We are beginning to explore why not passing a placement *feels* different from not passing other things.

Normally you have invested huge amounts personally and financially in becoming a health and social care professional. You will have a different relationship with your educator than you would with someone who marked an exam or a driving examiner. You will also have to go back out into the work area straight after receiving feedback that you have failed, often to face other professionals who are aware of what has happened and have often fed into your assessment. And unlike many other 'tests' you have to go into placement the next day having absorbed all the feedback and perform, when all you want to do is have a small or indeed large screaming fit about the unfairness of it all.

We hope you have identified some of those things mentioned above and possibly some different ones of your own. After all, failing is an individual experience but there are many common issues. Hopefully this chapter, in conjunction with support from your tutor from university and your educator, will support you through a fail on placement or help to reduce the anxiety for the people who have not failed but have turned to this chapter first!

Thoughts and feelings

There is no escaping the fact that hearing that you are not passing on placement feels horrible (we are being very polite here!). It seems to hot wire straight into the emotional side of your brain, often because you are aware that things are not going well and so your adrenalin is already pumping around your body and you are in 'fight or flight' mode. This often erupts in either anger or tears, which is normal.

As this chapter aims to support you through a fail it is essential that you get in touch with those feelings. This is not intended to be some new age psycho babble, it is a necessity because in order to move on, you have to acknowledge what you feel, relay this to others, hopefully in a controlled way and explore a way to move forward.

Imagine you are an actress or actor, this is the scene you need to play: you are in a supervision session, and your educator is sitting opposite you with the assessment booklet on a low table between you. You look at your educator and hear them say, 'I have to tell you that at this point in the placement you are not passing.' Obviously, if you are currently failing you can re-enact your own supervision session in your head.

We know everyone hates role play but remember that you are doing this on your own and for a reason. Also, you do not have to actually act it out, just write a list of your feelings once you have closed your eyes and imagined the scenario. How does hearing that information make you feel? Try to get in touch with some of those feelings and write a few ideas down in box 12.2.

Box 12.2

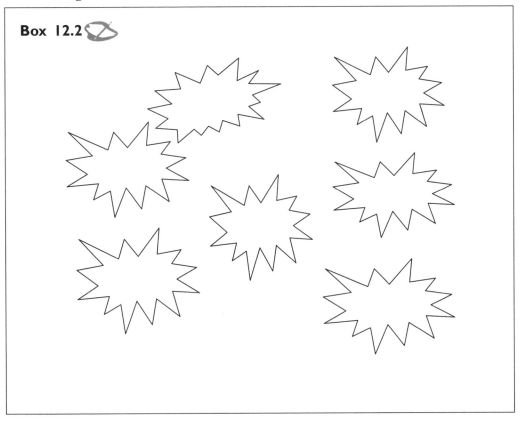

Here are some thoughts we have had. How do they compare to yours?

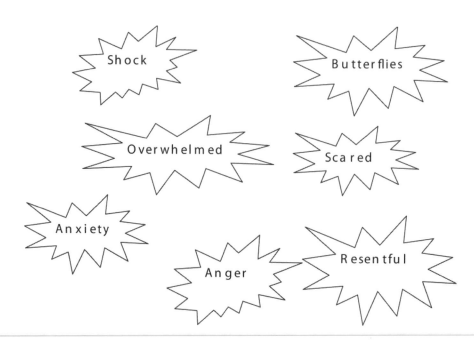

Looking at the combination of all of the above feelings go back to each burst of emotion, and identify what feelings could be constructive (tick sign) and which would be destructive (cross sign) to your future development.

While not disregarding your feelings, we think that it would be fair to say that out of all the above, you could talk about all of them with your educator (apart from any feelings of anger and resentment towards your educator!) The choice is yours, of course, but being angry and resentful are the hardest feelings to move forward from. Remember you have to come in again to the placement tomorrow and demonstrate your personal and professional development to the educator who is assessing you.

It is worth exploring why you feel angry and resentful, as often these feelings arise from a sense of unfairness or injustice. It may have some resonance with other times when the actions of parents or teachers have resulted in you feeling this way. Only you will know this and it is worth taking some time to think about this.

Before you continue, if this applies to you do get these feelings out of your system by writing them all down in box 12.3. Use your reflective journal and Chapter 3 on reflection to think things through. Try to talk to your university tutor or a friend.

Box 12.3 ⬲

The thing I find most unjust/unfair is
*

*

*

There may be many reasons why you may feel that your fail grade is not a fair reflection on your performance.

➡ 'My educator wasn't around when x happened.'
➡ 'I didn't know I couldn't text in if I was sick.'
➡ 'I just forgot to sign on the white board.'
➡ 'I didn't realise I was doing the initial assessment.'
➡ 'I thought I was just observing.'

To get the facts straight, it is your educator who makes the final decision about whether you will pass or fail a placement. That decision is not a personal decision about how you are as a person but about whether or not you have reached the minimum standard set for the level that you are at. Do not forget that you will have equal access to the criteria that your educator is using to assess whether or not you are competent. You should be familiar with your assessment form and the criteria on it should form the basis of your personal objectives. Try to be realistic about your own performance. Remember that it is not about the amount of effort you have made, it is about meeting the validated professional criteria.

It is very unusual that your educator would make the decision about whether you pass or fail alone. We do not say this to make you paranoid but instead to put the whole thing into some kind of perspective. Also bear in mind that telling another member of staff how unfair the whole thing is may backfire, as they may have contributed to the discussion about you with your educator before your supervision session. All these issues need to be offloaded to your visiting tutor from the university. You can use this visit to explore some of the issues that you have personally and professionally with the placement and possibly with your educator. Your liaison tutor can act as a third party to negotiate a potential path through some of the issues, and review your learning objectives with you.

Unless you can leave behind the majority of feelings of being unfair you will find it very difficult, almost impossible, to prepare for the coming week. You need to make some major decisions before you continue.

Failing at the halfway point – what now?

It is at this point in your professional career you will need to seriously evaluate your situation and try to work out what is most important to you at this moment in time. The final decision is yours and only you can make that decision.

Box 12.4

To help you come to a decision ask yourself some questions:

Why did I come on the course in the first place?

Think long and hard about this one as often this is where the answer about continuing or leaving the course is found.

Are all those reasons still valid?

Yes ☐   No ☐

If not what has changed?

Are there other things in my life which have come along since I started the course which seem to be more important?

➡ Have my priorities changed during the course?
➡ Is there something happening in my personal life which means that I cannot give this placement my full attention?
➡ Do I need some time off to sort out and then I can give my full attention to the placement?

And finally the most important question of all:

What decision would make me the most happiest when I wake up tomorrow morning?

Be as honest as you can when thinking about and writing the answers to these questions as it will help you to focus on your future personal and professional development. There are no wrong answers! Sometimes leaving the course is the best thing that you will ever do. Many people decide that the career that they have chosen is not as they thought it would be or that they do not enjoy the work, and this decision is usually made when they are on placement.

One other thing also needs exploring: *Is it you?* For whatever reason, things have changed and you may find that you do not actually want to do this career any more. Some people, for instance, discover on placement that they actually do not like working with patients/service users either on a one-to-one basis or in a group. You will need to think about this. There is nothing wrong with feeling like this but the health and social care courses are different from a history or sociology degree in that the placement is a taster of what you will be doing for a living. It will be your chosen career. If you feel ambivalent about people and you do not enjoy spending a lot of time with them and are not particularly interested in talking to them and finding out about how they are, this will affect your motivation and enthusiasm, something that will be picked up quickly by the staff around you. Most health care professionals are passionate about the client group that they work with, despite the politics and any general moaning. They are expecting you to be passionate or at least interested and will always express concerns about students who appear disinterested or unmotivated.

Is it the current placement area?

Sometimes it can just be the particular client/patient group that you are working with on this placement that you are not enjoying. There is evidence to show that certain personality types are attracted to particular areas of practice, and so some areas will immediately feel much more comfortable and you will feel 'at home' in them. Suffice to say that other areas will evoke the complete opposite feelings. However, for most people whichever area they are in, the client/patient group remains the focus of their placement and they concentrate on the skills that they are acquiring and their transferable skills. To work in health and social care you have to enjoy working with most people that you come across, and working as part of a team. Is that what you enjoy? If so, would you be better suited in another placement area? Did you come on to the course with an idea of the area that you would like to work in? Has your current placement got a faster or slower pace than you would like? Even if your current placement is not in an area that you would like to work in eventually there is still a great deal to be gained. Think about arranging visits and tutorials, explore your communication skills, build up a knowledge base that is transferable to an area that you would like to work in; in short, you will have to create your own motivation to succeed on the placement. If you can not think of an area that you would like to work in, then do not think of this as a failed placement but as an opportunity to review and reflect upon what you would like to do.

Finally, I am sorry to tell you at this point that 'not getting on with your educator' is not a reason for leaving a placement and has to be managed. But more about that later.

By this point you should have a 'gut' feeling about whether you would like to:

➡ continue with the placement
➡ I have a few days off to 'sort some things out'
➡ withdraw from the placement on the grounds of ill health
➡ withdraw from the placement because you have failed to meet the minimum standard required at this level, but are motivated to work towards a resit as this is the career for you
➡ withdraw from the course.

Whatever your decision, you must discuss all your options with your educator and your visiting liaison tutor to ensure that you receive all the relevant information that is available to you, about deferring, retrieval, credit points, etc. This will ensure you are making a decision based an all the facts and your own feelings.

Whatever your decision, well done on making it. It is not easy but you can be proud that you examined all the facts and feelings, reflected on them and made the right decision for you at this moment in time. If you have decided to continue with the placement you may wish to explore some of the possible issues in more depth.

What if I don't get on with my placement educator?

This is often a worry for first-time students and, 'What if I don't get on with my student' is equally discussed by first-time educators. Sadly as ever, there is not an easy answer to this. I hope throughout this book you have a taste of our honesty about placements and, to be frank, not getting on is not an option you have.

Throughout life there are many people that we have to be with that, given the option, we would not spend time with, we maybe related to them or have to work with them. We do not want you to write down their names but just think of one or two people from your past who may fall into this category. How did you deal with them?

If you have not written anything in the above space go back and try to think what you could do. Do not worry because different things work for different people; we will look at strategies together that you can use to enable you to work with someone that you would rather not spend time with. You may have already developed strategies, and if so fantastic. This is a chance to try them out again, reflect on them and evaluate them in a professional setting.

This is a great opportunity for your personal and professional development and one which you can grasp with both hands. Do not forget you will also have to work with clients and carers that you find difficult to deal with, so it is an invaluable skill. Here are some suggestions of strategies you can use. See if you can add to these suggestions and check how many match your own list:

❶ Put it on the agenda for supervision and ask your educator how they deal with difficult clients.
❷ Arrange visits to other areas.
❸ Try to identify some common ground, there is always something you have in common, if you think laterally and deeply enough, even if it is parking trouble or an interest in travel or a TV programme. It is worth noting here that you are looking for something to agree on, not something to increase any animosity!
❹ Remember the old adage about walking in someone's shoes. Try to have some empathy, for instance, think about what might be going on in their life? They might be thinking, 'I've got all this and a student to deal with!' Not everyone loves having students, and sometimes it just adds to the workload. Try the exercise in the Chapter 3 on reflection, this will enable you to explore a situation from another person's point of view and can offer many new insights and may make you view the situation more objectively than personally.
❺ Try to remain pleasant and positive, using phrases like: 'Thanks for that feedback, I can try and work on that.' We know it might be tough, but we did not say it was going to be easy!
❻ Silently analyse them. Try to work out why they behave in the way that they do. If nothing else it makes the whole situation more objective and interesting.
❼ Find out exactly how your educator wants you to behave during a supervision session, and then do it! You can worry about your principles after you have got through this placement!

I am sure you can think of many more, but if all else fails then be strong, check your behaviour constantly, remember why you came on the course and count the days down to the end of placement.

Many people fail a placement at the halfway stage and go on to successfully pass the next placement, using some of the strategies we have outlined. Students can also fail the placement but then go on to successfully pass the resit placement. If you are in this situation you need to receive clear feedback from your educator, and listen to this. You need to discuss your next placement with your university liaison tutor and think carefully about all the areas covered in this book. Each placement is an opportunity for a new start.

Initially, receiving this kind of news halfway through the placement can be devastating, but you have to listen carefully to your formative feedback and act upon it. You may feel that it is unfair or unjust but your educator has the final say and needs to explain fully to you and the university why you have not met the criteria. Do not forget that you have equal access to those criteria/competencies on your assessment form.

As we stated earlier many people fail at the formative halfway stage and then go on to pass the placement. This can happen for a number of reasons, which may apply to you. Maybe they did not know quite what was expected of them and then once told got on with it and demonstrated to the educator that they could reach the minimum standard required to pass. There may have been issues at home that have been resolved or it may have meant living in different accommodation if it is available and doing less travelling so that there is a little more energy for the placement.

All the options at the formative assessment can be discussed with your educator and university liaison tutor. You will need to take the responsibility even on your first placement and offer to go away and think about what has been said to you, reflect on this, and develop learning objectives for the rest of the placement. These revised objectives should clearly address the areas that you have failed in. If you have not done so already, now is a good time to work through Chapter 3 on reflection and identify why *you* think you have failed to meet the criteria, go through this with a fine toothcomb.

Take your objectives and some of your reflections with you into the next supervision session, or earlier if possible, to demonstrate that you have taken on board the feedback, have ownership of the behaviour and have identified clear ways that you can show your educator how you can achieve the minimum standards on the assessment form.

If you fail at both the formative and summative stages of placement then you will find yourself at a crossroads. If this is the formative halfway assessment you could go on to pass the placement. If this is the final summative assessment but your first fail, you will normally be able to do a resit placement.

At halfway or final assessment you always have choices that are open to you. These are:

➡ You could decide to continue with the placement if you are at the formative stage and try to pass, using some of the strategies we have discussed. At least you will be gaining more practice experience and giving yourself the opportunity to explore your own thoughts and feelings about the placement and career choice.

➡ You could decide, as many students do, that you wish to leave the placement at this point. This needs to be discussed with your educator and liaison tutor from the university to explore the options open to you, and the implications of your decision.

Failing the resit

For students who have already failed a placement, then this section of the chapter is for you because this is also an opportunity for reflection and a new start.

So what happens if after all this effort you have failed the placement? Sometimes you may have to face an unpalatable truth that this is not the career for you. This is always difficult, especially when you feel that you have given your all and there was nothing else that you could have done. We have been present at many failed placements over the years and every single one has been thought through thoroughly, with many educators losing sleep about failing students. It is not something that is entered into lightly; in fact, the easy option is to pass the student. Students unfortunately can fail placements for many different reasons. These include:

➡ poor communication skills
➡ lack of motivation and enthusiasm
➡ inability to problem solve
➡ limited academic ability
➡ inability to link theory with practice.

If you have failed you need to work through Chapter 3 on reflection and analyse what has gone wrong. This will involve exploring your own issues and not just blaming the educator/placement. If you find this difficult, then working as a professional in health and social care may not be for you at this moment in time.

Sadly, the assessments are not awarded for effort alone, as there are professional standards which must be adhered to, but if you have given your all to this placement then you need to be proud of your accomplishments, reflect on the placement experience with your educator and liaison tutor from the university and make a decision about where you would like to go to from here.

Failing a resit placement will ultimately mean that you have failed the course. If you are failing your second resit despite your best efforts, the hard truth is that this is not the right time for you to become a professional. This does not mean that the door is closed forever but that you may need more experience, a chance to sort out your personal life, or discover what you really want to do. If this course *is* what you want to do, you will need to go away and tackle the areas that have been identified and carry out the advice that you have been given, and re-apply in a couple of years.

For everyone who fails there is an opportunity to stop and rethink where they are going and what they want to do or are able to do. It is difficult in this scenario not to resort to clichés, but sometimes they can help you to think things through and move on. Write down a few to see if they can move you to a more positive place.

Box 12.5

If clichés do nothing for you, then write instead anything that would be valuable to you, 'If I have only learnt one thing from this experience it is.' Remember, there are many ways to solve a problem, if you do not like what you are offered, devise your own strategy, one that works for you.

We have been a third party in many failed placements and although difficult at the time, it is always an opportunity for you to explore complex issues and enable you to move forward in whichever direction you ultimately choose. It is vital that you use this chance of reflection in a positive way to enable you to move forward. Whatever happens you will have learnt some invaluable lessons about yourself, your strengths and the areas that require more working/reflection on. Ultimately, you will learn far more from your mistakes (although this is not always immediately apparent), especially if you can put the experience behind you and move on and you owe it to yourself to do just that.

Chapter outcomes

Now that you have completed this chapter you should feel more confident to:

➡ explore failure objectively
➡ identify your thoughts and feelings around failure and its implications for your future personal and professional development
➡ work out objectively whether this is the right time and place for you to continue with the placement
➡ prepare for your supervision sessions and halfway/final report.

Well done on completing this chapter – it is a difficult one.

Further reading:

Maxwell, J. (2000) *Failing forward: turning mistakes into stepping stones.* Thomas Nelson Inc.

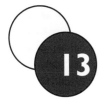

13 Not quite the end …

- **Rewarding yourself**
- **Moving on**

At the end of this chapter you will be able to:

➡ review your developments
➡ identify what you have enjoyed and what you have struggled with
➡ Reflect on these areas
➡ give yourself a pat on the back
➡ write a timed action plan.

Well done, you have almost finished this book. We hope you have enjoyed working through the exercises and they have given you some food for thought.

At the beginning of this book we talked about continuing personal and professional development. Even though you have finished working through this book you will have realized by now that the journey of a professional does not end unless you stop being a professional. As long as you are working with people you will need to review and reflect on what you are doing in order to offer the patients/clients the best possible service.

Box 13.1

By now you should be feeling fully prepared for your placement.

Have a look at the list below. Think about what you have done and what you have achieved while working through this book. Award yourself a tick for every chapter completed, decide on your own reward system for each tick.

Preparing personally for placement	
Reflecting on your behaviour	
Participating in supervision	
Self-assessment	
Writing learning outcomes	

Making complex decisions using your professional reasoning skills	
Work/life balance and time management	
Knowledge of working with other professionals – where you fit in the jigsaw	
Keeping a record of your progress personally and professionally (portfolios and progress files)	
Evidence-based practice	

Well done! Giving yourself a pat on the back every now and then is essential. We hope you have enjoyed your reward, even if it was only ten minutes of daydreaming!

You have worked through a great deal of material, which should enhance your personal and professional development. Do not worry if there are a few areas that need more work. Sometimes that work never ends but being aware of it is an important development in your levels of insight into your own behaviour. No one is expecting you to be perfect and indeed none of us are or ever will achieve that accolade. However, it is important to be aware of where your strengths are and the areas which you are working on, especially if you are working as part of a team. It will also help when you have supervision. Remember that you have come on the course to learn and are not expected to know everything. You only need to demonstrate what you do know and how you are going to achieve all the areas that you will be assessed on.

Here is a list of the chapters in this book. Now you have worked through this book you will have used a wide range of self-ranking scales, you can decide how to rank the work that you have enjoyed the most using a score or a description in box 13.2. Maybe you could try using some of the ratings with your client/patient group? If you asked them to evaluate their treatment, having explained what the evaluation is and what you will be using it for, of course.

Box 13.2 ⊘

Enjoyed? Struggled?

Preparing personally for placement	
Reflecting on your behaviour	
Participating in supervision	
Self-assessment	
Writing learning outcomes	
Making complex decisions using your professional reasoning skills	
Work/life balance and time management	
Knowledge of working with other professionals – where you fit in the jigsaw	
Keeping a record of your progress personally and professionally (portfolios and progress files)	
Using evidence-based practice	

Now that you have assessed yourself you need to do some analysis. Reflect on each chapter and why you struggled with it or why it was easier or more enjoyable:

(?) How does this link with your developments on placement?

(?) How does this link with your development on the course?

This information can be used in your progress files or CPD (continuing professional development) file. It demonstrates your developments during the course or placement and could act as a baseline for evidence of developments in the future.

Rewarding yourself

As we have said throughout this book, becoming a professional and obtaining state registration is not easy. You need to reward yourself when you have worked hard at a piece of work. Sometimes those rewards will be small – a cup of tea or coffee at the end of a chapter, going out with friends after the completion of an assignment – and sometimes major reward, such as a holiday at the end of a year or the end of a course. It is vital that you acknowledge that you need a pat on the back. In completing this book you need to give yourself a reward, however small, to recognize the work that you have done and what you have achieved. It would obviously be good to hear this from someone else. On your course you will receive written or verbal feedback on your assignments. On placement you will receive feedback during supervision sessions but in both areas the tendency is to listen for and focus on the areas in which you are not doing very well. Try to balance that out and allow yourself to listen for the things that you have done well and acknowledge those strengths. In supervision if you feel things are not balanced ask for this matter to be put on your agenda if you are not hearing anything positive.

Here are just some of the skills you should have when you have completed one or more placements:

➡ By now you should be able to prepare for placement and think through some scenarios before you encounter them.
➡ When working with clients you will be able to make complex decisions using your professional reasoning.
➡ When incidents happen on placement you should have the skills to reflect critically on the experiences and identify a range of critical incidents which you can evidence in your portfolio.
➡ You should be able to self-assess using your own university assessment form and then identify areas which you need to work on.
➡ Writing learning objectives which are SMART will demonstrate clearly how you are going to achieve the objectives you have set, the timescale, and the right level for you.
➡ You will be able to negotiate the agenda for supervision and discuss the areas that you are working on using your objectives to illustrate this.
➡ Listening to feedback you will be aware of the balance of positive and negative and use it constructively to review your developments.
➡ Underpinning all this is your understanding of team work and the value and role of other members of the interprofessional team.
➡ You will be aware of the importance your developments but also ensure that you have a good work/life balance using your developing time management skills.

Moving on

It is now time to move on! You have worked hard and hopefully achieved a great deal. You may be going back to university now to continue with the course or you may be ready to graduate and are looking for a job. Whatever your next step is you will need a plan to keep you focused and motivated. Using all the skills that you have developed throughout this book you will need to write yourself an action plan in box 13.3 for the next three months. You may want to discuss it with your educator or personal tutor or use it as evidence in your portfolio.

Box 13.3 My action Plan

Action   Date

Action	Date
1.	
2.	
3.	
4.	
5.	

And now, a final well done! Thanks for working through this book. We hope you have found it useful.

Chapter outcomes

Now that you have completed this chapter you should have:

➡ reviewed your developments
➡ identified what you have enjoyed and what you have struggled with
➡ reflected on these areas
➡ given yourself a pat on the back, or some other reward
➡ written a timed action plan.

Well done! You have completed this final chapter. Good luck for wherever life takes you.

Index